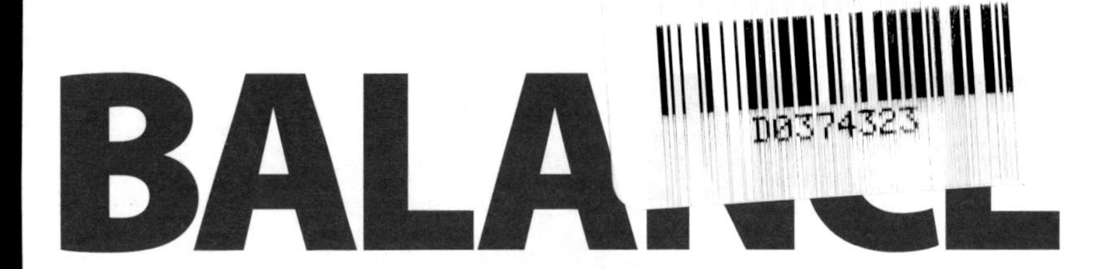

A guide for managing dental caries for patients and practitioners

2nd Edition

V. Kim Kutsch, DMD
Robert J. Bowers

www.balancebook.com

Bill Blatchford, DDS
President and CEO, Blatchford Solutions

BALANCE — A small book with a large message. Drs. Kutsch and Robert Bowers have nailed the opportunity to change the lives of your patients. This could be the most significant change in dentistry as we know it. This changes the dentist from fixing the results of disease to actually curing disease. Make a difference by doing things differently. Two thumbs up.

Bruce B Baird, DDS
CEO, Productive Dentist Academy

The book educates any dentist on the cause and effect of dental caries and the disease process. It is a must read for all dentists. After 33 years it has changed the way I approach diagnosis and treatment planning.

Gary Hutton, DDS

I requested a copy of ***BALANCE*** *as an opportunity to compare the text's offering with the CAMBRA program currently in use in my office. The material is well presented. The one item which we do not utilize routinely is the ATP caries screening; otherwise I am pleased that our program is in line with the texts plan; re-enforcing our efforts as solid when creating our program two plus years ago. The organized and structured approach to caries and periodontal risk assessment has motivated our hygiene department; patients have become much more engaged in their care; and their compliance has contributed to their improved overall health, and better dentistry. It is much more enjoyable to be able to provide restorative care when the tissues are healthier. Hygienists and patients are also tickled that zero bleeding on probing is achievable as part of the program.*

I also like the reasonable/cautionary approach advocated by the authors regarding the use of probiotics. I agree that correction of the pH dysfunction is a necessary precursor to their use. So many advocate probiotic use without necessarily being founded in good science.

Kurt S Black, DDS

Timberhill Dental has been practicing CAMBRA and dispensing CariFree product since its introduction to the profession and we thought we had a pretty good grasp of the whole picture … till we read ***BALANCE****. Wow, that book got the entire practice buzzing and has clearly outlined why and how to apply the CariFree line of chemotherapeutic treatment products. A recommended read if your practice is committed to this new standard of care.*

Christine Taxin
President, Links2Success

As an adjunct professor at NYU Dental School, I will be recommending this book to all students. As a speaker around the country I will continue my personal quest to bring the home care information to the doctors and teams I meet. We should all take the wonderful information, the products that can help and continue our co-diagnosis with our patients and the medical community so the light of health can shine bright.

Nancy Cheung, RDH, MPA/HSA

BALANCE — ***A guide for managing dental caries for patients and practitioners*** *is a book every dental professional should have. It's comprehensive and contains a wealth of information. The graphics, layout and organization of the book, patient examples are excellent. I will definitely be incorporating this book into one of my courses in the dental hygiene program.*

Albert Clark, DDS

BALANCE is, as it claims on the cover, "a guide for managing dental caries" and it is an excellent one. However, it is much more. Containing case histories, scientific studies , excellent charts and illustrations, It not only outlines a system to manage caries, it in simple terms explains the balance that defines the caries process, and invites the reader to explore a new paradigm of dental care. We have watched the development of Dr. Kutsch's approach for three to four years and have witnessed the benefit to our patients. It just gets better and better. Thank you Kim!

This book can be read in an evening or studied for days. You owe it to yourself and your patients to explore its contents.

Brent Ingram, DDS

As a dentist, I am always looking for ways to explain to patients plain sense ways of my prevention program I have been using in my office for over 20 years. The information contained this book does just that. Thank you.

Thimy Le, DMD

The book was amazing. I was able to sit down in the chair with my patient and show them what I was talking about and actually explain to them what they can do. It was very informative but simple to understand.

Allison Boatright, RDH

When my team started utilizing this program for our patients, I was excited to provide the best care for managing dental caries. Each chapter in the book taught me something new. I especially enjoyed the chapter regarding patient examples. This chapter answered most of the questions I had. It gave me insight to some of the same issues my own patients were dealing with. This book is the perfect guide for any team member to provide information and answers to any dental caries question they may have.

Linda Lukacs, DDS

*Whether you are a dental professional, dental student or a patient, **BALANCE** is an easy to read, easy to understand, review of the process of dental caries and risk assessment. The paradigm shift from dental treatment to dental prevention is refreshing. While this book appeared very simple at first, it provides a comprehensive overview on the pathology of caries, methods to identify those patients at greatest risk for tooth decay, and strategies aimed at prevention.*

Susan Mclearan, RDHAP, MS

I very much enjoyed the book. Having followed Dr. Featherstone for quite some time and having participated in our ECC education program here in California, the book provides a clear look at the critical factors that should be addressed. It was a good read and I am sharing it in any way I can.

Patti DiGangi, RDH, BS
Speaker, author, clinician

Dr. Kutsch and Mr. Bowers deliver in the slim, impactful book an amazingly credible definition of the new paradigm for caries management. This isn't the newest version of how to sell dentistry or fix teeth and gums. Each of the chapters clearly takes readers through the steps of CAMBRA-caries management by risk assessment from understanding the disease process, identifying and understanding specific risk factors to creating individualized plans with patients. The book paints a strategy for success for both patients and practitioners by including case studies, insurance benefit coding and the science behind the philosophy.

As with all great works, it reads simply and conveys complex concepts in a way any reader can grasp. I personally read book cover to cover yet it is just as accessible to be read non-linearly. This book should be on the shelf of every dental professional. The public should also read it so they can help 'push' the profession toward change.

Mr. Richard Celko Aetna's National Dental Director of Utilization Management said in 2009, "The nation's largest dental carriers (Aetna, BCBS, CIGNA, Delta, MetLife, etc.) have been tracking their internal data for years. The preponderance of evidence suggests that it makes more economical sense to the patient, insurance carrier, and the employer purchasing the plan to pay for prevention rather than paying for the restoration or extraction of teeth. As a result, some of the nation's largest dental plans are covering more preventive and diagnostic services in hopes of avoiding more costly and invasive restorative services in the future." Balance gives practitioners the definitive guide to create this future.

Debi Gerger, RDH, MPH

A fabulous guide for managing dental caries allowing all dental professional to ascertain their role in risk assessment and the associated patient care. Dental Hygiene educators should consider this book as part of the cariology curriculum as it provides science, therapy based on risk level, and patient case studies.

Pat Pine, RDH

*After reading the book **BALANCE** — I felt every oral health care professional should have this reference in there offices. I found that it reached out and showed professionals what is necessary to get a balance to our patients. I feel pH testing is underused in dentistry. This is an avenue that dentistry has ignored and should embrace.*

*Many are about the bottom line — ph testing is about the patient oral and physical health. It tells a story. Any dental practice can help their patients with MI Dentistry. MI Dentistry is here, it will not go away. Less invasive dentistry is as important as less invasive medical care. Patients have not connected oral and physical health — I feel it's moving slowly. Balance, it's all about balance in our lives. Reading the book was a great eye opener for me — I am already a believer in MI Dentistry and **BALANCE**. This book shares so much information that all professionals should have at their fingertips.*

Mike Nelson, DDS

*I have been a dentist for over 30 years. **BALANCE** is at the foundation of a paradigm shift in the way we understand the tooth decay/caries process. Whether a dental professional or a patient (and in reality, we are all patients) **BALANCE** will give you an appreciation as to WHY some people get decay more than others and HOW to manage and halt the decay process.*

*When I was in dental school, decay was battled with a toothbrush and floss. Today, and since 2007's landmark research on CAMBRA (CAries Management by Risk Assessment) dental caries is taught to be a communicable disease. Preventing caries requires understanding and managing diet, saliva, AND bacteria. Brushing and flossing still remain foundational tools in our fight, but if you still get cavities, after reading **BALANCE** you will understand the missing link in your battle.*

*I have given this book to the hygienists, periodontists, and orthodontic offices that I work with. I now believe that dental caries need never exist, and if it does exist, need never progress. Bold statement? Is it easy? If you value the investment you have made in your oral health, **BALANCE** will teach you how to protect those pearly whites.*

Paul Brannen, DMD

*As dentistry moves further from the surgical, "drill and fill" model of treating decay and closer to the treatment of dental caries as a disease, it can sometimes be difficult to make sense of it all. For new dentists who may not have been taught this treatment approach in dental school, or experienced dentists who are interesting in staying on the cutting edge of dentistry today, **BALANCE** provides a systematic, evidence-based approach to the treatment and prevention of dental caries as a disease and delivers the message in an easy-to-read, easy-to-understand book that takes little more than an evening or two of reading to complete.*

*As a public health dentist that works in an area with some of the highest dental caries rates in the United States, I'm keenly aware of the dental caries epidemic today. Consequently, dental caries management is the cornerstone of any public health dental clinic. **BALANCE** has proved invaluable in our clinic that employs multiple dental providers from many different educational backgrounds and treatment philosophies. It allows us to provide them with a clear, concise reference of our dental clinic's treatment approach and has resulted in consistent, predictable dental caries management for our patients.*

I highly recommend this book to anyone that is interested in providing lifetime dental health to their patients, their family or themselves.

Ryan Speirs, DMD

*I am most of the way through reading **BALANCE**. I've found that the concepts around caries management are laid out in a manner that is easy to understand and supported by research from sources that dental professionals know and trust. The idea of shifting to a more preventative model gets me excited about the restorative care that might be avoided if oral imbalance is properly managed.*

ISBN: 978-1-60594-964-2 (PB)
978-1-60594-965-9 (EB)

Published by Llumina Press
Second Edition

Library of Congress Control Number: 2012915294

This book is dedicated to our families, who have encouraged and supported us throughout the process.

Thank you.

Acknowledgments

The authors would like to acknowledge the following individuals (in alphabetical order) who have inspired them with their leadership, research, and commitment to the field of dentistry and dental prevention. Without leaders like them, this book would never have been possible.

Robert F. Barkley, DDS
John B. Featherstone, MSc, PhD
Margherita Fontana, DDS, PhD
Kerrod B. Hallett, BDSc (Hons), MDSc, MPH, FRACDS, FICD
Edwina Kidd, BDS, FDS, PhD, DSc
John C. Kois, DMD
Tom J. Maier
Curtis A. Machida, PhD
Philip D. Marsh, BSc, PhD
Graeme Milicich, BDs
David Noel, DDS, MPH
Brian B. Novy, DDS
Francisco Ramos-Gomez, DDS, MPH, MS
Douglas A. Young, DDS, MS, MBA

A special thank-you to the dentists and dental teams that participated in the private practice research study.

Dr. Mary Kingery, Kingery & Kingery
Dr. Brian Roberts, Ash & Roberts DDS
Dr. Steve Ash, Ash & Roberts DDS
Dr. Michael Young, Forever Young Dentistry
Dr. Sean Rockwell, Rockwell Family Dental

Foreword

John D.B. Featherstone, MSc, PhD
Dean and Professor
School of Dentistry, University of California San Francisco

Publication of this book is a major step forward in the implementation of "caries management by risk assessment" (CAMBRA) that will change the face of dentistry and lead to reductions in dental caries such as we have not seen since the advent of fluoridated drinking water and fluoride toothpaste. This is a must read for every hygienist, dental assistant, general dentist, as well as every dental specialist. The disease we call dental caries is an issue for all. For example, the prosthodontists who are attempting to deal with ongoing decay in high risk individuals in whom they have done wonderful reconstruction work. This book provides straightforward messaging to help in a very practical way to provide dramatically better oral health for individuals.

I have been involved with caries related research for almost 40 years. About 25 years ago it became very obvious that translation of what we knew into every day practice would likely take decades to accomplish, while at the same time we would continue to learn more about the science of the disease. In 1999, when I first published the concept of the "caries balance" my naïve hope was that this would immediately translate into reductions in dental caries in everyday dental practice. However, it was not to be. The balance concept is so simple and grew out of the demineralization/remineralization "tug of war" idea of the 1980s. All diseases in the body progress or halt depending on the balance between pathological and protective factors, so why should dental caries be any different.

In the early 2000s the California Dental Association Foundation supported our efforts to provide peer reviewed published materials for the practitioner and auxiliaries to use with patients every day. These publications and all the people who got "on board" started the CAMBRA activities and now there are many new and effective products, written directions, forms, outcomes assessments, and a growing body of evidence supporting what started as a dream based upon the then-available science. Very exciting progress has been made over the last 10 years. With the advent of the present publication, “Balance” there is no further excuse for practitioners and auxiliaries to ignore what is becoming the standard of care. Intervention and preventive therapy based upon risk assessment and necessary minimally invasive restorations to follow sums it all up in one sentence.

I challenge everyone who reads this book to put the concepts into practice and be part of the paradigm shift in the treatment and management of dental caries.

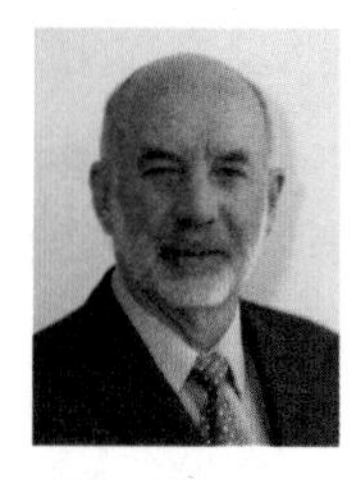

Professor John Featherstone is Dean of the School of Dentistry at the University of California, San Francisco (UCSF) and Professor of Preventive and Restorative Dental Sciences. He holds a Ph.D. in chemistry from the University of Wellington (New Zealand). His research over the past 38 years has covered all aspects of cariology (study of tooth decay) as well as laser effects on dental hard tissues. He has received numerous National and International awards, including the Norton Ross Award for excellence in clinical research from the American Dental Association (2007) and is an Honorary Fellow of the American College of Dentists. He has published over 240 papers and book chapters.

Douglas A. Young, DDS, MS, MBA

Ever wonder why some people continue to get cavities despite efforts by the dental team, while others do not? A healthy mouth requires more than brushing, flossing, and "fillings." Dental caries, and the subsequent dental decay, is a complicated multifactorial disease of epidemic levels affecting children and adults. *Balance* addresses current trends in caries disease management, including caries risk assessment, new detection technologies, and therapeutic strategies for managing this disease. With the current scientific evidence and new technologies, patients and practitioners can begin to look at caries from not just a purely restorative (drilling and placing fillings) approach but also a medical (preventive/therapeutic) approach. This information allows patients and their dental specialists to select proper therapeutic strategies designed to prevent, stop, or reverse the cavity process.

Caries risk assessment is evolving into the best practice of care in dentistry. Identifying the disease indicators as well as the pathogenic and protective factors specific to each individual is an essential component in managing a patient's oral health. This moves the dental profession's approach to management of dental caries from a "drilling and filling" treatment model to a healing model. *Balance* is an excellent guide for managing dental caries that belongs in each and every dental practice and should be read by any patient seeking a dental home or considering a restorative treatment.

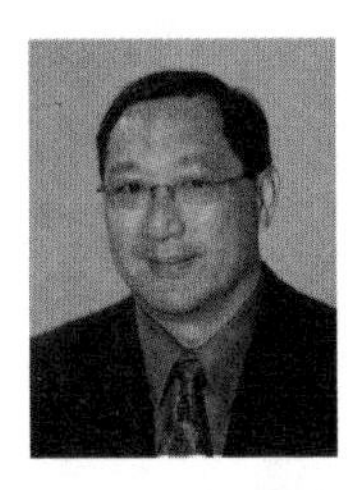

Dr. Young is an active and ardent educator in the field of minimally invasive dentistry, dental materials, and cariology. He serves on several boards and has presented at congresses around the world, including the World Clinical Laser Institute, the Academy of Laser Dentistry, the World Congress of Minimal Invasive Dentistry, and several universities. He has also been published in several peer-reviewed dental journals and textbooks. In addition to speaking and publishing, he also conducts extensive research on minimal

invasive dentistry, lasers, and cariology. He has performed clinical trials using lasers, as well as studying caries inhibition by laser irradiation, and optical caries detection technologies. He is an associate professor at the University of the Pacific and an associate clinical professor, adjunct, at the University of California–San Francisco. He is currently active in teaching clinical dentistry to the students at UOP and research at UCSF.

Contents

Introduction

There are many myths surrounding the cause of cavities, and maybe you have heard a few. "Maybe you just have soft teeth." "Sugar causes cavities." "Just brushing and flossing twice a day will prevent cavities." "Fillings will stop the decay process." "You can't 'catch a cavity' from someone else." "Fluoride is a conspiracy, and it doesn't actually help prevent cavities."

While some of these sayings are partially based on facts, and some are simply not true, actual research exists and reveals the truth. Cavities, also known as dental caries, are caused by a bacterial imbalance on the teeth. This imbalance occurs based on each individual's oral environment, dietary habits, and hygiene habits. By understanding what causes an imbalance in the oral environment, and by making adjustments, the bacterial imbalance can be controlled and a patient's cavity rate can be either reduced or eliminated. The goal of this book is to provide both patients and practitioners with a guide to help identify issues a patient may face, and the range of potential treatment strategies a patient may choose in order to improve their oral health and keep their teeth for life.

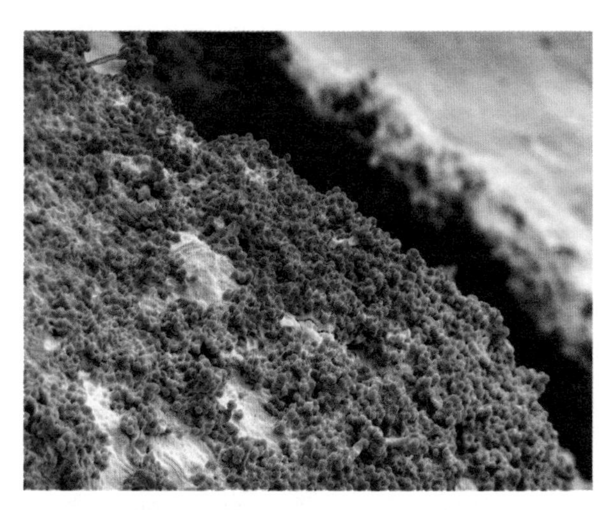

Bacterial biofilm and red blood cells on the teeth

According to the CDC (Centers for Disease Control and Prevention), dental caries is an epidemic in the United States; and although it is largely preventable, it remains the most common chronic disease of children aged 5 to 17 years—4 times more common than asthma (42% versus 9.5%). According to the CDC in the US population,

- 28% of children aged 2–5 have already had decay in their primary (baby) teeth;
- 50% of children have experienced tooth decay by age 11;
- 68% of 19-year-olds have experienced tooth decay in their permanent teeth—more than two-thirds;
- low-income children are twice as likely to experience decay as children of higher-income families.
- 52,000,000 school hours are lost each year due to dental disease;
- much of the dental disease in both children and adults go untreated;
- 16% of children aged 6–19 years have untreated dental caries;
- 23% of adults aged 20–64 years have untreated dental caries;
- most adults will experience dental disease, and many will lose teeth;
- 85% of all adults experience tooth decay;[1] and
- more than 60% of adults will lose a permanent tooth due to cavities.[2]

According to the American Dental Association and the American Academy of Pediatric Dentistry, the new dental standard of care for managing a patient's risk and preventing dental disease is to perform an individual "caries risk assessment" analysis during dental appointments. Dental disease (caries) today is best assessed, diagnosed, and managed by identifying disease indicators and risk factors, and examining the balance between pathogenic and protective risk factors.[3,4,5,6,7] This process provides both patients and practitioners with specific future decay risk probability that is specific to each patient. Patients found to be at risk can then be presented early intervention advice, educational materials, and prescription/professional therapies.

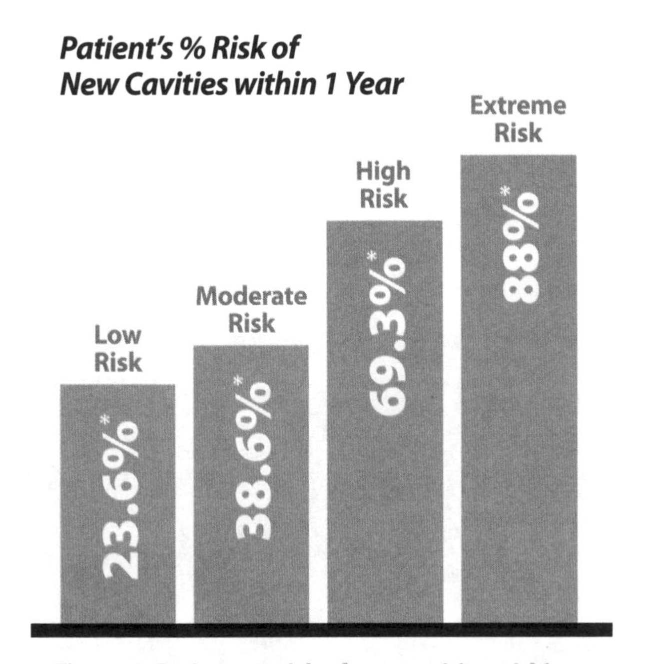

Figure 1. Patients % risk of new cavities within 1 year based on caries risk

S. Domejean, J. White, and J Featherstone, "Validation of the CDA CAMBRA Caries Risk Assessment—A Six Year Retrospective Study," *Journal of the CDA*, (October 2011):714.

Everyone with teeth is at some form of risk for the infection that causes decay. Based on a major population study of close to 13,000 patients, even low-risk individuals have a 23.6 % chance of developing new cavities in the next 12 months. Conversely, high/extreme-risk patients have an 88% chance of developing new cavities in the next 12 months (See Figure 1). Patients can lower their risk by choosing to change some of their lifestyle habits, change their dental home care program and the products they use, and regularly visit their dental professional to monitor progress. The process of caries risk assessment in the private dental practice was first introduced in 2003, and published and

...published and unpublished studies have shown that caries risk assessment, along with early-intervention professional products, can lower decay rates anywhere from 25% to 74%.[8]

unpublished studies have shown that caries risk assessment, along with early-intervention professional products, can lower decay rates anywhere from 24% to 74%.[8] For some patients, this means a reduction in their decay rate from 10 new cavities per year down to fewer than 3. Some patients with nonmodifiable caries risk factors may only experience a limited benefit, but for many, it means a lifetime of being cavity or decay free.

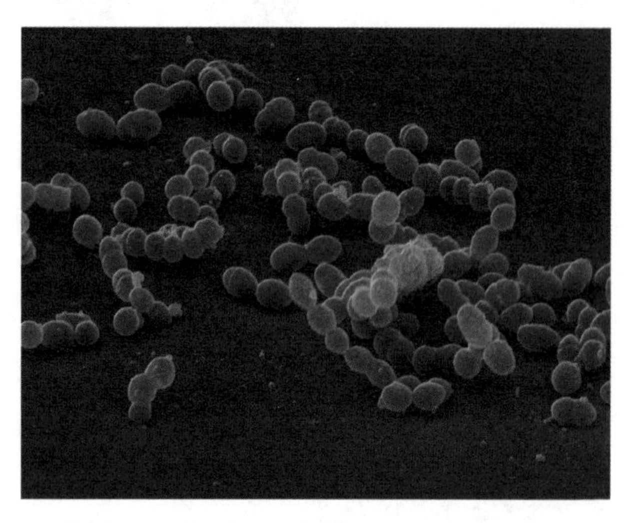

Cavity-causing bacteria, *Streptococcus mutans*
© Eye of Science/Photo Researchers, Inc.

Unfortunately, there is no "silver bullet," "magic pill," "guarantee," or "vaccine" for dental decay; and educated dental professionals do not see one coming in the near future. Dental caries is a multifactorial, multiple-pathogen biofilm disease.[9] While some progress has been made in the immunization against *Streptococcus mutans* and genetically modified bacteria, typically, complex biofilm diseases do not respond readily to vaccines, antibiotics, or replacement therapies.[10] Not to mention the current dental caries disease model also includes potential systemic effects on the rest of your body from the disease. *Streptococcus mutans* (a cavity-causing bacterial species) is the most common oral bacteria found on heart valves and coronary arteries when it is found in the mouth of an individual.[11] This species has been demonstrated to invade artery lining tissues and may be responsible for infections in the heart and valves, bacterial endocarditis, and may also have other potential risks for heart diseases.[12] Other oral bacterial species that have been identified with dental caries may also play a role in other systemic infections and complications.[13] Every patient's oral bacterial profile is as specific to them as their own fingerprint, and the guidance of a trained dental professional is absolutely essential to their oral and overall health.[14]

Step 1:

Understand the Disease Process and How Cavities Form

Cavities are caused by the bacterial imbalance/infection known as "caries." Dental caries is a transmissible bacterial infection of the teeth that leads to net mineral loss in the teeth, resulting in white spot lesions, cavitation, and potential tooth loss. This disease is prevalent in all age groups and a chronic disease among many patients.[15] Historically, the disease model involved two primary pathogens, *Mutans streptococci* and *Lactobacillus;* however, additional pathogens are being identified every year, and some 40 different bacteria within the oral biofilm have now been implicated in this disease.[16, 17]

...dental caries is a pH dysfunction of the normal biofilm on the teeth.[18]

All humans have a small layer of bacteria on their teeth. This layer of bacteria is called a biofilm. A biofilm is a community of microorganisms meshed together in a sticky film, and caries is now understood to be a biofilm disease. In recent years, as our understanding of the complexity of biofilms has increased significantly, so has our appreciation for the complexity of this disease. Current biofilm studies suggest that dental caries is a pH dysfunction of the normal biofilm on the teeth.[18]

What this means is that prolonged periods of low (acidic) pH in the mouth provide the biologic oral environment that selects for the growth of cavity-causing bacteria and at the same time is responsible for the demineralization and net mineral loss of the teeth (See Figure 2).[19] The bacteria that play a role in dental caries are acidogenic and aciduric. This means that they produce acid as a by-product when they metabolize or digest food sources, and unlike healthy, desirable bacteria, they are uniquely adapted to live and thrive in an acidic environment. By producing lots of acid, they create an environment within the biofilm that does not allow for healthy bacteria to survive. Unfortunately, this acidic environment is also responsible for the breakdown of the tooth structure. This production of acidic conditions in the biofilm eventually creates a shift in the bacterial makeup, favoring more acidic bacteria, which results in yet more mineral loss on the teeth.[20]

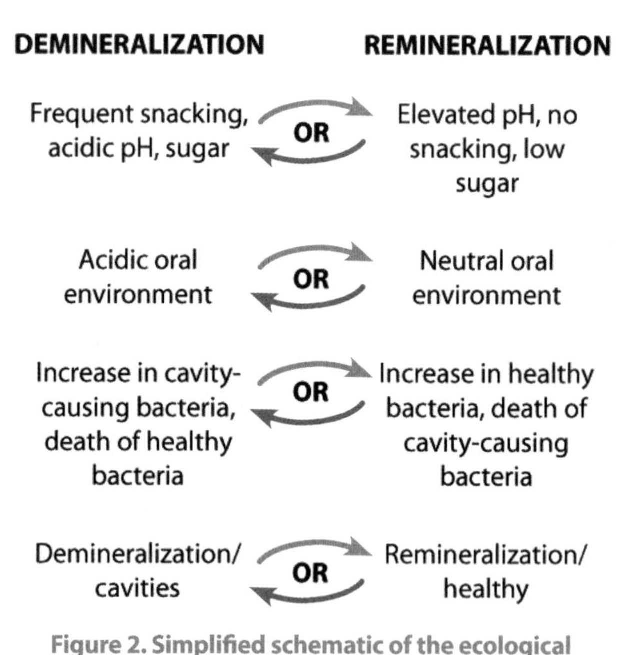

Figure 2. Simplified schematic of the ecological plaque hypothesis proven

(Philip Marsh, "Marsh Schematic of Ecological Plaque Hypothesis," *Oral Microbiology:* 116)

These cavity-causing bacteria in biofilms are strongly resistant to antibodies, antibiotics, and antimicrobial agents.[21] Consequently, biofilm diseases do not respond to surgery, vaccinations, or antibiotic/antibacterial strategies that target one species of bacteria. In order to effectively treat dental caries, not only must we restore the teeth to function, but the dental biofilm needs to be restored to health and the pH dysfunction corrected.[22]

Step 2:

How to Identify a Patient at Risk

In order to identify if a patient is at risk for cavities, the dental practitioner must identify if the patient has any risk factors for the disease dental caries. A risk factor is simply something that increases your risk for a disease. For example, smoking is a risk factor for lung cancer. Likewise, many risk factors have been identified for cavities.

The most common methods of identifying risk factors is to have a patient fill out a risk assessment form or have a dental practitioner interview a patient to assess their risk factors. This process of identifying a patient's risk for dental caries (the bacterial imbalance that causes cavities) is called CAMBRA.

The acronym CAMBRA stands for "CAries Management By Risk Assessment." CAMBRA is a method used by preventive dental practitioners for assessing caries risk and making dental treatment and restoration recommendations based on a patient's caries risk.

A simple comparison used to understand CAMBRA methodology is to compare it to a risk assessment for heart disease your physician may perform during a physical examination (See Figure 3).

Risk Factors for Heart Disease	Risk Factors for Caries
Heredity	*Current decay condition*
Age	*Current bacterial challenge*
Sex	*Decay history*
Tobacco usage	*Dietary habits*
Alcohol consumption	*Current daily medications*
Weight	*Saliva flow*
Dietary Habits	*Medical conditions*
Physical activity level	*Presence of oral appliances or braces*
Stress level	*Oral hygiene habits*
Other present disease conditions	

Figure 3. Comparison of risk factors for heart disease and risk factors for caries

When assessing risk for heart disease, a physician will perform tests for blood pressure and cholesterol count. Then they will examine and interview for other risk factors such as heredity, age, sex, tobacco usage, alcohol consumption, weight, dietary habits, physical activity level, stress level, and other present disease conditions.

The physician will then make recommendations based on the above risk factors. For example, patients with a low-level risk for heart disease may be good candidates for running a marathon or having any elective cosmetic surgery. On the contrary, patients with a high-level risk for heart disease may not be good candidates for running a marathon or having elective surgery and may require medical intervention such as prescription medications or diet and exercise counseling.

Dental professionals who perform CAMBRA are performing a similar function. Based on risk factors for caries disease, dental professionals will perform tests for oral bacteria levels as well as take x-rays and perform a thorough oral examination. They will then examine disease indicators and risk factors such as current decay condition, current bacterial challenge, decay history, dietary habits, current daily medications, saliva flow, medical conditions, presence of oral appliances or braces, and oral hygiene habits.

Patients at high risk may require medical intervention in the form of prescription / professional oral rinses, gels, gums and sprays.

The dental professional can then make recommendations based on the above risk factors. Patients at high risk may require medical intervention in the form of prescription/ professional oral rinses, gels, gums, and sprays. They will also require restoration of any existing tooth decay. High-risk patients may also receive recommendations to put off elective cosmetic dental procedures, whitening, or orthodontics until risk levels can be decreased. Patients at low risk may receive recommendations for home care preventive oral products to keep risk levels low and will be better candidates for elective cosmetic dental procedures.

Patients who are assessed as high risk are more likely to have failures in expensive dental work due to recurrent decay. The challenge for dental professionals is that the patients who have the highest need for restorative care also come with the highest risk for restoration failure. Studies have shown that high/extreme-risk patients have an 88% chance of new decay within the next 12 months.[23] The dental professional performing CAMBRA will include treating the cavity-causing bacterial infection/imbalance and risk factor recommendations in addition to the restoration treatment plan based on the patient's specific risk factors to reduce the risk of restoration or cosmetic failure due to recurrent decay.

Many dental journals have been dedicated to the subject of CAMBRA, and CAMBRA methodologies, like heart disease risk assessment, have proven to reduce decay rates in all age groups. The *Journal of the California Dental Association* dedicated their February and March 2003, October and November 2007, and October and November 2011 journals to CAMBRA.

It is extremely important to mention that having risk factors identified does not mean an individual has current cavities, or that an individual is guaranteed to have cavities in the future. Just as a physician may identify a risk factor for heart disease, it does not mean that a patient is guaranteed to have a heart attack; simply there is a greater risk. Risk factors are identified in order to get a clear picture of what the likelihood is patients may experience dental disease in the future, and to provide practitioners with evidence-based information and the ability to target therapeutic recommendations to each individual patient and decrease their risk of future disease signs and symptoms.

Step 3:

Understand the Specific Risk Factors for Caries

While a number of risk factors for caries that ultimately lead to cavities will be covered in this section, there are four primary risk areas that are often the root causes of dental disease: bacterial biofilm imbalance/infection, poor saliva/inadequate saliva flow, frequent snacking/acidic drinks/destructive diet, and poor home care/wrong home care product routine. Experienced CAMBRA clinicians can often point one, two, or all of these primary risks as the causes of a patient's dental decay. While each will be covered in detail, it is important to note that the severity of a patient's risk and the resulting signs/symptoms of decay increase when multiple risk factors are involved.

Bacterial Biofilm Imbalance: Bad Plaque and/or Too Much Plaque

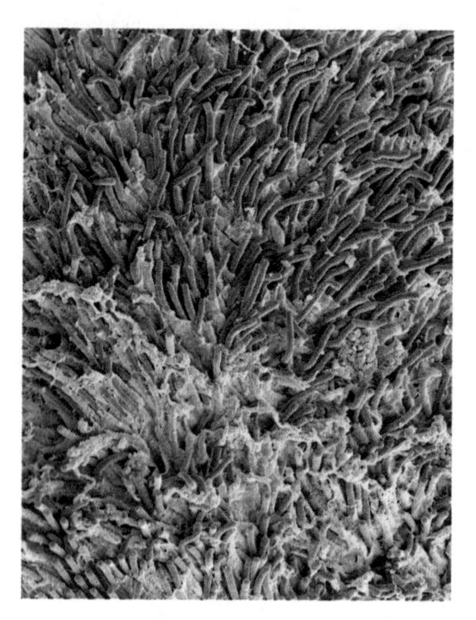

Dental plaque biofilm
© Eye of Science/Photo Researchers, Inc.

The bacterial biofilm on teeth discussed earlier is commonly referred to as dental plaque. Dental plaque consists of a community of diverse bacteria from more than 700–800 different species of bacteria.[24] While there is great diversity in the potential bacterial makeup of any given patient's dental plaque, typically, a healthy person has only about 120 different species in their dental plaque. Interestingly, patients with high risk for dental caries may have more gross amount of plaque but usually have fewer total species.[25] Not as many bacteria are adapted to survive in the low pH conditions of the dental-caries-producing plaque or biofilm. Dental plaque is a risk factor for cavities primarily in two different ways. First, if the plaque biofilm on your teeth has a high concentration of the cavity-causing bacteria (acidogenic/aciduric), there is an increased risk of tooth mineral loss. Second, if there is too much total bacterial plaque on your teeth, there is an increased risk of tooth mineral loss.

The growth and type of dental plaque biofilm can be influenced by several factors, including the availability of nutrients, the pH of the oral environment, and the roughness of the tooth surface as rougher surfaces present an ideal setting for microbial adhesion.

There are many ways to identify if a patient has too much plaque as a risk factor. First, if a patient or practitioner notices any visible plaque buildup between brushings. Plaque buildup between brushings is a sign of a highly active biofilm, and the bacteria within the biofilm are reproducing quickly.

Additionally, a dental professional can perform a plaque index check which can gauge the degree of dental plaque accumulation. This is done by providing the patient with a plaque-disclosing dye solution that will color all of the tooth surfaces containing plaque. The practitioner will then count the number of plaque-containing tooth surfaces and divide it by the number of available tooth surfaces. For example, if a patient has a total of 100 tooth surfaces and 70 are identified as containing plaque, the patient's plaque index is 70%. There are numerous plaque indices that have been used over the years in dentistry.[26] However, they are time-consuming and not many dental practices perform a routine plaque index check.

A dental professional can also perform a bacterial ATP swab test or bacterial culture to identify patients who have a prevalence of the cavity-causing bacteria in their dental plaque as well as a high bacterial load.

In order to perform a culture test, a patient must supply a saliva sample, which is then cultured to identify the quantity of bacteria in the mouth. Currently, culture testing is only commercially available for 2 of the 40+ strains of cavity-causing bacteria, and the culture requires 48–72 hours to incubate before results can be identified. Studies have also demonstrated that these cultures do not provide an accurate assessment of the levels of bacteria being cultured and are not predictive of dental caries. Due to the high cost and long time required for culture testing, few dental practices perform it.

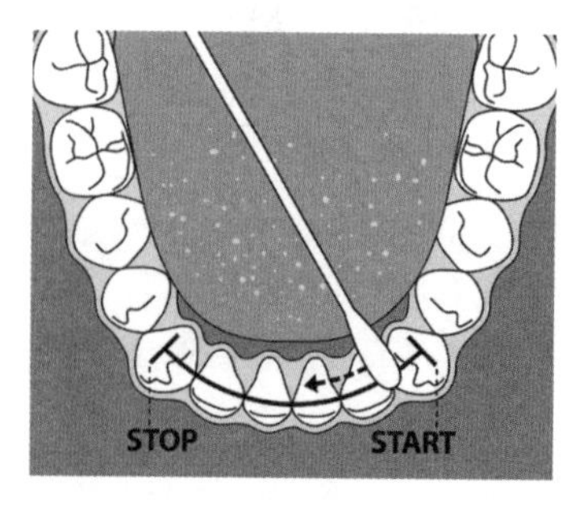

Figure 4. Example of area swabbed in CariScreen Test

The dental professional can also opt to perform a bacterial ATP CariScreen swab test (See Figure 4). This swab test is a quick, painless procedure, and results can be identified in less than one minute. ATP is often used for caries risk screening as high numbers of ATP correlate to both high quantities of bacteria in the dental plaque and high quantities of cavity-causing bacteria in the dental plaque. Bacterial ATP screening is a good indicator of future decay and is not used to assist in diagnosing current decay. Not all dental practices perform CariScreen testing.

A patient is at risk if they have too much plaque buildup/accumulation, or a high quantity of cavity-causing bacteria within their dental biofilm. This risk factor is commonly referred to as biofilm challenge and/or plaque buildup. Patients that are found to have high volumes of bacterial plaque or high numbers of cavity-causing bacteria in their plaque may be recommended a professional broad-spectrum antibacterial therapy, pH neutralization products, xylitol-containing products, and increased fluoride exposure to reduce the biofilm challenge.

Dry Mouth/Saliva

Saliva is one of the most important protective mechanisms of the teeth. It contains proline-rich proteins and glycoproteins, mucins, calcium, phosphate, and bicarbonate, along with a host of other antibacterial, antiviral, and antifungal constituents. Saliva performs many functions, including assisting in food digestion, protecting the body from microbes, balancing the pH in the mouth, and supporting the remineralization of teeth.[27] The body maintains the hypermineralized structures (teeth) by continually bathing them with a supersaturated solution of tooth mineral.[9] Without saliva, teeth would simply dissolve.

Due to saliva's protective functions, a lack of saliva, often referred to as dry mouth or, more technically, xerostomia, is a major risk factor for dental disease.[23, 29] Consequently, it is a risk factor question when a dental practitioner discusses a patient's dental caries risk.

Studies have shown that dry mouth affects 20%–46% of the total population.

Everyone, at some point in his or her life, suffers from dry mouth.[27] But a significant feature of dry mouth is that it occurs in women more often than in men; it is also more prevalent among older adults than in young or middle-aged individuals, is usually more severe during sleep when salivary glands naturally produce less saliva, and can occur due to many factors. While only a small percentage of patients self-report symptoms of dry mouth, studies have shown that dry mouth affects 20%–46% of the total population.[27]

Some of the causes of dry mouth are stress, poor diet, age, heredity, disease, and commonly used medications that cause dry mouth as a side effect.

There are a few ways to identify if a patient does not have enough saliva and has "dry mouth" as a risk factor. First, if any in the following list of common dry mouth questions occurs occasionally or more often during the day, a healthy dry mouth relief therapy should be investigated:

Some of the causes of dry mouth are stress, poor diet, age, heredity, disease, and commonly used medications that cause dry mouth as a side effect.

1. My mouth feels dry.
2. I notice a lack of saliva in my mouth.
3. I get up at night to drink.
4. My mouth feels dry when eating a meal.
5. I have difficulties swallowing certain foods.
6. I sip liquids to aid in swallowing foods.
7. I suck on sweets or cough drops to relieve dry mouth.
8. My throat feels dry.
9. My mouth becomes dry when speaking.
10. I regularly use ______ to keep my mouth moist.

Another method of identifying dry mouth is the resting or stimulated saliva flow test.

For the resting saliva test, the dental practitioner may ask a patient to spit into a measuring cup without any oral stimulation for one minute and then assess the amount of saliva. If the resting saliva flow is less than 0.1ml/min, it is very low, 0.1–0.25ml/min is low, and 0.25–0.35ml/min is normal.

For the stimulated saliva test, the dental practitioner may ask a patient to spit into a measuring cup while chewing on a piece of sterile wax for five minutes. If the stimulated saliva flow is less than 0.7ml/min, it is very low or high risk, 0.7–1.0ml/min is low, and 1–3ml/min is normal.

Many dental practitioners can also identify upon oral inspection if there is a saliva/dry mouth issue present. Another simple test is resting saliva flow, which averages about 0.3 ml/min. The practitioner can retract the lower lip and observe saliva droplets forming on the mucosa of the lip from the minor salivary glands found there. Within a minute, there should be numerous droplets of saliva. Another quick indication for saliva flow is to just look at the floor of the mouth. The body produces about 1 liter of saliva every day, and a healthy patient will have saliva pooling at the floor of the mouth. Not all dental practices, however, perform saliva testing.

Medications That Cause Dry Mouth

Dry mouth is an underrecognized but common side effect of thousands of over-the-counter medications, prescription medications, and dietary supplements. Due to the dramatic effect low saliva flow or poor saliva quality has on the oral health of patients, particularly increasing caries risk, the American Dental Association (ADA) commissioned a letter in April 2011 to the commissioner of the Food and Drug Administration (FDA) as well as the director of Center for Drug Evaluation and Research. In this letter, the ADA respectfully requested that the FDA consider requiring medications that are commonly associated with dry mouth side effects to carry warning-label information about the oral complications associated with reduced salivary flow. The letter specifically stated, "Without the cleansing effects of saliva, chronic *[medication induced]* dry mouth can lead to tooth decay."[29]

Without the cleansing effects of saliva, chronic [medicated induced] dry mouth can lead to tooth decay.[29]

For this reason, it is important to share any and all over-the-counter medications, prescription medications, and dietary supplements with your dental professional. Many of the most commonly prescribed medications are associated with dry mouth, including analgesics (pain medications), antidepressants, antihypertensives, acid reflux medications, seizure disorder medications, and antianxiety medications. Other common over-the-counter medications like analgesics (pain medications), allergy medications, antihistamines, and decongestant/cold medicines can also cause dry mouth.[30] Dry mouth has also been reported by patients taking oral contraceptives and vitamins/dietary supplements.[31]

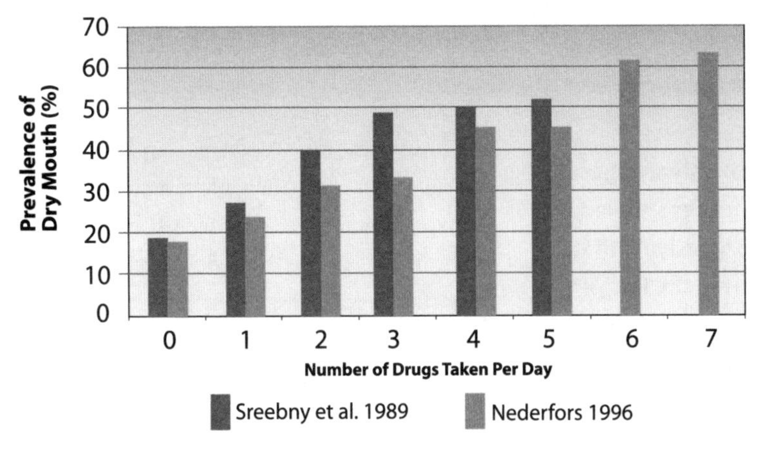

Figure 5. Prevalence of dry mouth based on number of drugs taken per day

T. Nederfors, "Xerostomia: Prevalence and Pharmacotherapy, with Special Reference to Beta-adrenreceptor Antagonists," *Swed Dent* J 116, Suppl (1996): 1–70.
L.M. Sreebny, A. Valdini, and A. Yu, "Xerostomia. Part II: Relationship to Nonoral Symptoms, Drugs And Diseases," *Oral Surg Oral Med Oral Pathol* 68 (1989): 419–427.

While each and every patient responds to medications differently, data taken on all drug consumptions, including all prescription drugs, OTC preparations, and alternative drugs, clearly shows that the prevalence of dry mouth increases with the number of drugs taken every day. As much as 20%–30% of patients taking just 1 drug daily report dry mouth. This progressively increases to greater than 60% when 6 or more different drugs are taken daily. Alternatively, less than 20% of people who do not take any drugs complain of oral dryness. This indicates that even the removal of a single drug, regardless of its dry mouth potential, may help reduce the incidence of dry mouth (See Figure 5).[32]

Unfortunately for many patients, their daily medications may be an unmodifiable risk factor. Especially among the elderly, patients are generally taking multiple drugs to combat life-threatening diseases. It is not recommended to stop taking any prescribed medication without consulting the prescribing physician. For those who cannot remove medications from their diet, there are alternatives, such as saliva replacements, pH neutralization products, xylitol-containing dental products, and increased fluoride exposure.

Drinks and Snacking (Diet)

Collectively, these studies showed conclusively that it was the low pH generated from sugar metabolism rather than sugar availability that led to the breakdown of microbial homeostasis in dental plaque.[36]

Every time we eat or drink, the pH in the mouth becomes acidic. The more often individuals eat and drink, the more frequently the pH becomes acidic in the mouth, giving the cavity-causing bacteria an opportunity to thrive.[19] Our bodies are designed to defend against this pH drop by secreting more saliva. Saliva is designed to buffer the pH back up to healthy levels. The pH of resting saliva is 6.75, while the pH of stimulated saliva is 7.8 to help the mouth recover from the drinking/eating episode. There are also bacteria in a healthy biofilm that function to help raise the pH back to healthy levels immediately following an acidic period. As the pH drops during the drinking/eating episode, when it gets below a pH of 5.5, small amounts of tooth mineral dissolve from the teeth and are trapped in the biofilm on the surface of the teeth. In a healthy mouth, within 15–30 minutes of drinking/eating, the pH recovers and raises above 5.5, and this mineral then returns to the teeth. When the system is in balance, the pH drops, some mineral is lost from the teeth, the pH recovers, and the mineral returns to the teeth. When the system is out of balance, prolonged periods of low pH cause net mineral loss from the teeth. The constant pH balancing act in the mouth has a direct effect on a patient's risk for cavities, and often is the most common cause of increased dental caries.

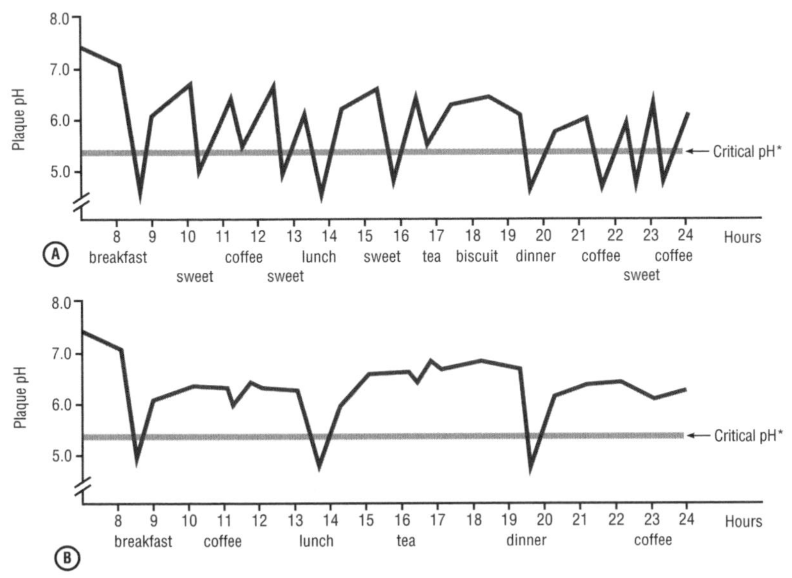

Figure 6. Schematic representation of the changes in plaque pH in an individual who (A) has frequent food and drink intake during the day, or (B) limits their food and drink intake to main meals only. The critical pH is 5.5, below which teeth begin to demineralize.

Marsh, Philip D., Martin, Michael V., *Oral Microbiology;* 12.

In order to determine whether what a patient drinks or their dietary habits could be contributing to their caries risk, two questions are asked during a caries risk assessment and near-verbatim questions have been validated in university-based trials. These questions are primarily focused on identifying frequency of consumption and oral exposure rather than what type of food and drink the patient is consuming.

1. Do you drink liquids other than water more than 2 times daily between meals?
2. Do you snack daily between meals?

To maintain a low-risk status, one should eat and/or drink four to five times daily as their daily limit of food and beverage (other than water) intake. As a patient increases the frequency of exposure to food and drink, they are increasing the number of acid attacks their teeth experience.[35] The more acid attacks a patient experiences, the more likely the patient's biofilm will change from normal healthy bacteria to cavity-causing bacteria, and their teeth are also experiencing demineralization during the acid attacks.[35] Frequent snacking and drinking liquids other than water (including alcohol, which can cause dry mouth) can have a profound effect on a patient's caries risk.

One area that often becomes a question is the "speed" at which food and drinks are consumed. From a caries-risk standpoint, it is much better to drink three sodas at one meal than to sip on one soda continuously for several hours (See Figure 7). If a patient is going to consume sugary snacks or drinks, it is better to do it during a standard mealtime or consume it quickly to allow their saliva to return their oral biofilm to a healthy pH level. Patients that take small

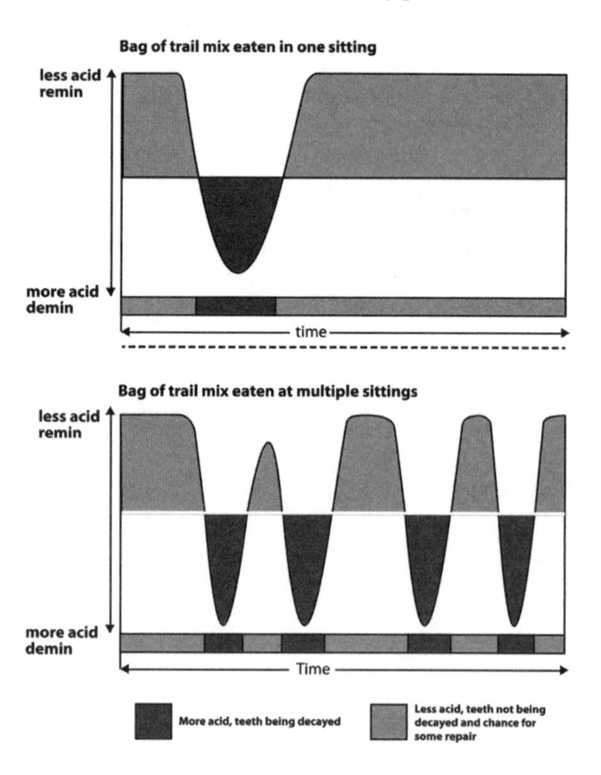

Figure 7.

bites of food or sip on beverages over long periods are not giving their oral environment and biofilm the chance to return to a healthier pH level. Ideally, sugary or acidic foods and drinks should be limited as part of a healthy diet if a patient wants to lower their incidence of cavities or their risk of cavities in the future.

For many patients, it is tough for practitioners to explain the increase in caries risk due to frequency of eating and drinking to patients who either "only snack on healthy foods" or are on a frequent meal diet. While frequently snacking on healthy foods or being on a frequent meal diet may be better than snacking on sugary foods or helps improve the patient's waistline, it does increase a patient's risk for cavities.

For some patients, their diet is strictly controlled for health reasons, or they are not willing to make dietary changes at this time. For these patients, dental products exist in the forms of gums and sprays that can elevate the pH in the mouth immediately after a food or drink acid attack and contain xylitol, which is a natural sweetener that reduces the growth and acid production of cavity-causing bacteria. Using these products regularly can reduce the risk of cavity-causing bacteria taking over a patient's biofilm and causing cavities.

Poor Home Care/Wrong Home Care Product Routine

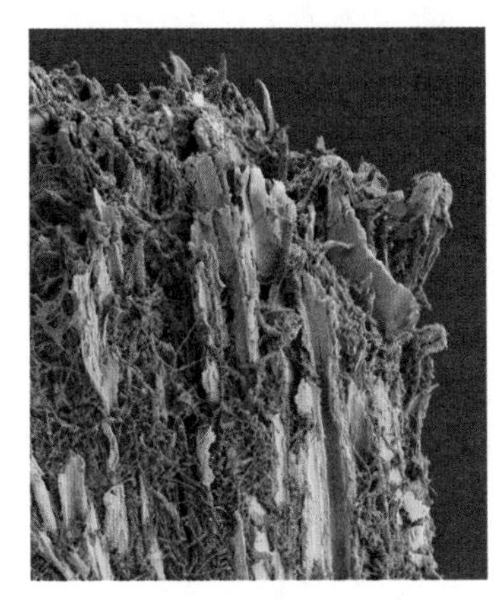

Dental plaque on a used toothpick

Many individuals have been taught since they were children to "brush and floss your teeth twice a day to keep the dentist away."

While this is excellent advice, and removing food debris and some of the plaque buildup from your teeth is important, it does create one question: how many infections/diseases are treated back to health with either a piece of string or a short handle plastic stick with bristles on the end? While mechanical removal of debris and plaque should not be ignored, the chemotherapeutic agents being brushed with, rinsed with, etc., are the actual therapy agents that have the ability to alter the oral biofilm and ultimately influence oral health. For example, a high/extreme-risk caries patient with severe decay, low saliva flow, and bacterial imbalance who has been regularly brushing and flossing is not going to suddenly get healthy if they increase their current brushing and flossing regimen from twice a day to 4 times a day. Simply put, if the products and home care routine they were using were working…well, it would have worked.

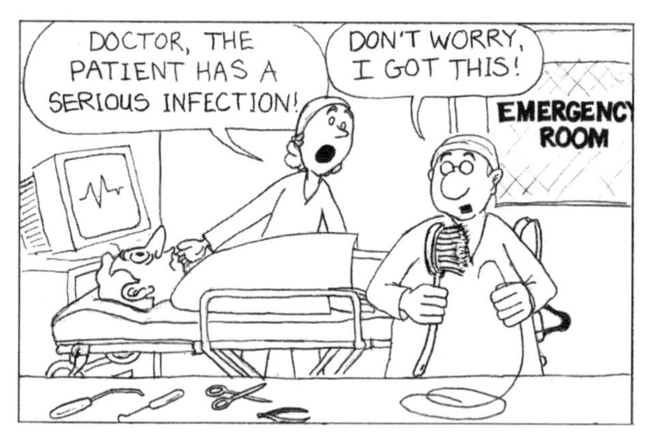

Can you really cure an infection with a brush and piece of string?

Most patients receive little to no guidance from their dental professionals regarding products they should be using at home, and the supermarket aisle is awash with products that can "do everything" and products that are "recommended by 4 out of 5 dentists." The most common advice routinely offered to dental patients is to "brush and floss more." For many patients, this advice can be frustrating, especially when they are already brushing and flossing regularly but still have cavities.

> **Most preventive dental practices that sell professional dental therapeutic products earn less than 1% of their annual revenue from product sales. If a dentist has chosen to carry and sell a product in their office, they have chosen it due to its potential to help their patients.**

On the other hand, offices that are serious about recommending proper patient-specific product therapies are often met with equal frustration from patients. These patients often mistakenly believe the practitioner is just trying to "push products to make money." The reality is that dental practices do not earn much, if any, profit from selling professional dental products, and few, if any, dental practices choose the products they wish to recommend to their patients based on "profitability." Most preventive dental practices that sell professional dental therapeutic products earn less than 1% of their annual revenue from product sales. If a dentist has chosen to carry and sell a product in their office, they have chosen it due to its potential to help their patients. Dental ethics prevents dental practitioners from "upselling" or "pushing" medical therapies on patients that are not indicated. If a patient has received a CAMBRA home care recommendation, it should be taken very seriously.

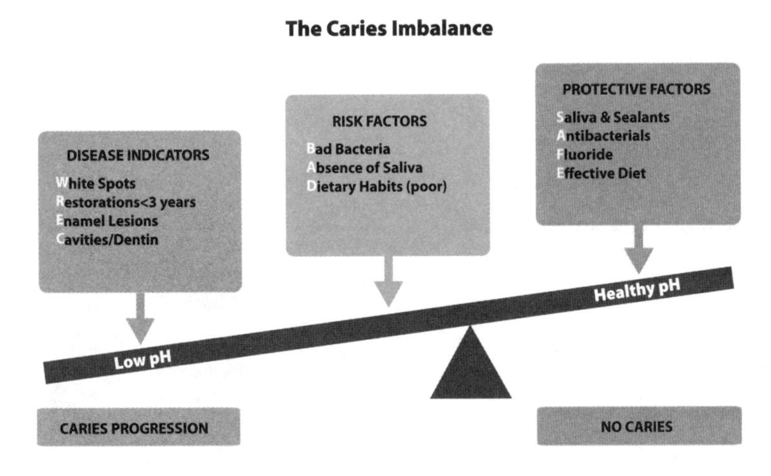

Figure 8. The Caries Imbalance – John B. Featherstone, MSc, PhD

J. B. Featherstone, S. Domejean, L. Jenson, M. Wolff, and D. Young, "Caries Risk Assessment in Practice for Age 6 Through Adult," *CDA Journal* 35, no. 10 (October 2007).

The balance among disease indicators, risk factors, and protective factors determines whether dental caries progresses, halts, or reverses. Dr. John Featherstone, of the University of California, San Francisco School of Dentistry, introduced the concept of the caries balance in 2002 while performing a caries risk assessment clinical trial on close to 13,000 patients. The concept and clinical trial have since been validated. In basic terms, in order to reverse the progression of dental caries, a patient must "outweigh" their disease indicators and risk factors with protective factors specific to their needs. For some patients, the disease progression is so great that it is a challenge to reverse the trend and can take substantial time and effort to tip the balance toward health.[33]

A proper home care program is simple. It is designed to counteract the risk factors specific to each patient with products the patient is willing to purchase and use as directed by their dental professional and weights their individual "caries balance" (See Figure 8) toward health. Unless there is a contraindication, the recommended products should contain some or all of the known caries therapy agents (See Figure 9) such as pH neutralization, therapeutic levels of xylitol and fluoride, remineralization agents like nanoparticles of hydroxyapatite, as well as a broad-spectrum oxidizing antibacterial agent if a biofilm imbalance exists. Other recommendations should include a reduction of all modifiable risk factors.

Oral Appliances

Oral appliances are not one of the most common risk factors, but many people do require the use of oral appliances throughout their lifetime. Oral appliance refers to braces and orthodontic brackets, orthodontic retainers, "clear braces" aligners, sports mouth guards, night guards, sleep apnea appliances, whitening trays, and partial dentures—basically, any type of foreign dental object placed in the mouth for an extended period of time.

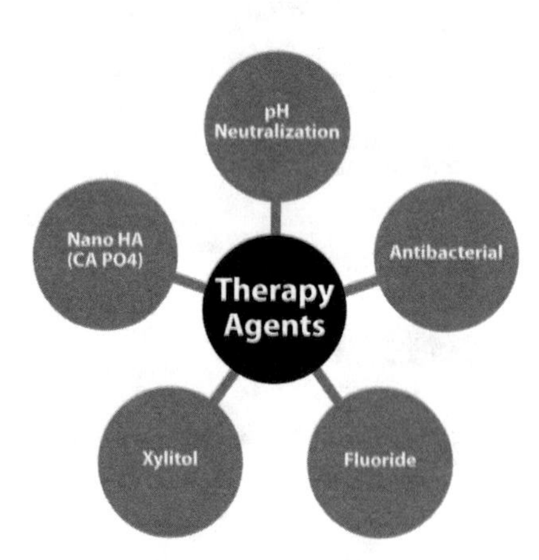

Figure 9. Five recommended therapy agents for high caries risk patients

Oral appliances are a risk factor for caries for two reasons: oral appliances can create artificial areas on the teeth that are much harder to keep clean and remove the cavity-causing bacterial plaque and food debris, and oral appliances create artificial zones on the teeth that limit the exposure to protective saliva flow.

One of the primary oral appliance risks is orthodontic braces. Studies have shown that 60.9% of patients with braces (average of 1.9 years' duration) experienced white spot lesions (tooth's enamel has taken on an opaque color in the area where cavities are beginning to form).[34]

Regardless of other risk factors, and the patient's present risk status, the high caries risk nature of these appliances for patients, especially braces, the dental professional should consider some form of additional prevention therapy such as pH neutralization, xylitol, nanohydroxyapatite for remineralization, and additional fluoride exposure. Oral rinses can be especially beneficial in assisting patients with oral appliances in delivering the therapeutic agents into hard-to-reach areas due to the appliance. Some patients with night guards, sleep apnea appliances, and clear aligners can also place small amounts of neutralizing therapeutic gels into the tray and wear them overnight for increased protection.

If a patient is considering using oral appliances, braces, or clear aligners for cosmetic tooth alignment, or any other oral appliance for a non-health-related issue such as whitening, it is recommended that the patient identify their caries risk status first. The patient may decide to delay cosmetic dental procedures until they are low or low/moderate risk prior to moving forward if white spot lesions and increased caries activity are a concern.

Other Health Concerns

Dental professionals will often also interview a patient for other health concerns as they may have an effect on the patient's saliva flow, acid exposure, or diet/food frequency.[33] Some of these health concerns are the following:

1. Frequent Tobacco Use
    a. Frequent tobacco use, particularly smoking, can cause dry mouth and reduced salivary flow.
2. Acid Reflux
    a. Patients with acid reflux can have stomach acids reflux into the throat or mouth regularly bathing the teeth with very low pH (pH 1.5–3.5) stomach acids. Patients with this condition may notice

a sour taste in their mouth and/or a burning sensation in their upper abdomen/chest.

b. Patients with acid reflux are also often taking over-the-counter or prescription acid reflux medications that cause dry mouth.

3. Diabetes

a. Individuals who are diabetic often have diet restrictions and eat many small meals and snacks sprinkled throughout the day in order to keep the amount of carbohydrates down at each meal. As a result, their blood sugar stays more balanced, which prevents high and low blood sugars. Conversely, the frequent eating/snacking in order to control blood sugar does not allow for their saliva to maintain a healthy pH level. For diabetics, diet is often an unmodifiable risk factor, and professional oral care therapies are frequently the best option for preventing or reversing a caries infection.

b. Dry mouth is also one of the most common oral health problems for diabetics; in many cases, it is due to medications prescribed for treating diabetes. The combined effect of frequent snacking and low saliva flow places individuals with diabetes at an increased level of risk for the caries infection.

4. Bulimia

a. Individuals with bulimia can have many issues placing them at greater risk for caries infection and tooth loss. Usually, dental professionals will notice acid erosion on the lingual surfaces of the maxillary incisors (back side of the upper front teeth) and on the mandibular incisors (lower front teeth) caused by the regular exposure to stomach acid. Beyond acid erosion, the regular acid challenge in the mouth can increase the likelihood of acidic bacteria overtaking the biofilm.

5. Head and Neck Radiation Therapy

    a. Radiotherapy for head and neck cancer results in severe and chronic salivary gland dysfunction in most individuals. This results in significant side effects, including dry mouth, difficulty swallowing, and malnutrition, which are linked to significant reductions in patients' quality of life and increased caries risk. Many patients going through head and neck radiation therapy have such a reduced volume of saliva flow that they literally can watch their teeth dissolve due to the accelerated caries rate. They pose a real challenge to the dentist as they are also at risk for postextraction osteoradionecrosis, where the bone does not heal following tooth extraction. In years past, many of these patients would have all of their teeth extracted prior to the radiation treatments. Today, with the advances in radiation treatment, and the ability to manage dental caries, most of these patients keep their teeth but are at significantly increased risk for decay, and the dental profession needs to monitor and manage their care closely.

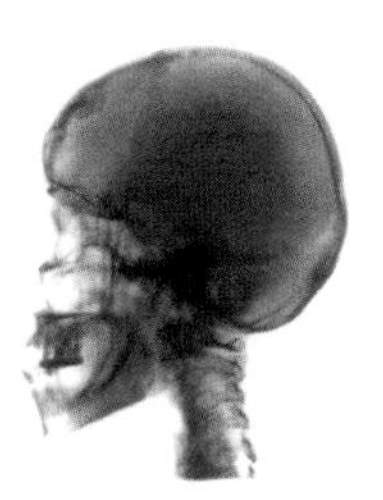

6. Sjögren's Syndrome

    a. Sjögren's syndrome is a chronic disorder of the immune system in which the patient's white blood cells attack the saliva and tear glands. This leads to dry mouth and eyes because the body's tear and saliva production is reduced. Many patients often don't know they have Sjögren's syndrome. Reaching a diagnosis can be difficult and generally takes an average of 6.5 years from the onset of symptoms to make the correct diagnosis. Part of the difficulty with diagnosing Sjögren's is that many of the symptoms, like dry mouth, mimic symptoms of other issues such as dry mouth caused by medications. Saliva substitutes are essential for patients with Sjögren's syndrome.

7. Other Drug Use

    a. While other drug use is often not something patients choose to discuss with their dental professionals, it is a risk factor for the disease and illicit drugs have severe oral health consequences. Other drug use includes drugs such as methamphetamine, marijuana, opiates/heroin, cocaine, ecstasy, and derivatives of such drugs like crack cocaine. The primary reason these drugs increase the risk for caries infection is the side effect of dramatic reduction in saliva flow. Many other drug users also commonly have a high caries-producing diet and frequent intake of carbonated beverages.

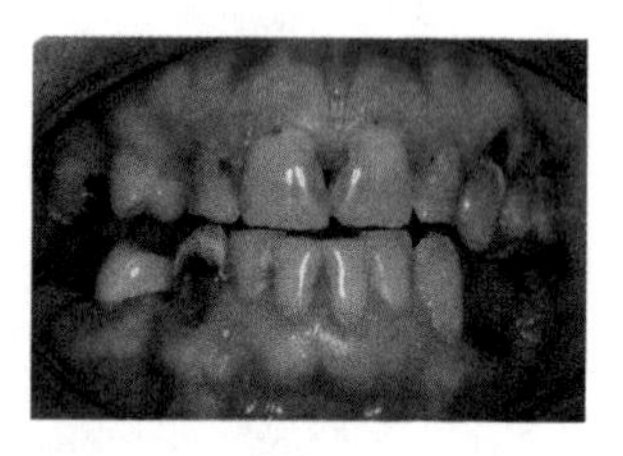

There is quite an extensive list of risk factors for caries, which ultimately leads to cavities. But as mentioned earlier, there are ultimately four primary risk areas that are typically the root causes of dental disease: bacterial biofilm imbalance/infection, poor saliva/inadequate saliva flow (which has many causes), frequent snacking/acidic drinks/poor diet, or simply the wrong home care product routine per the individual's risk factors. By identifying the specific issues facing each individual patient, dental professionals and patients can choose to make specific risk factor changes targeted uniquely to the patient's needs. These include behavioral changes and/or prescription/professional products designed specifically as *protective factors* to put the patient back on the road toward oral health.

Step 4:

Know Your Protective Factors and Agents

A simple definition of "protective factors" is that they are factors that weight patients toward health rather than disease. Just as a healthy diet and exercise are protective factors against heart disease, there are a number of "protective" therapy agents a patient can choose to correct an oral imbalance as well as protect themselves from an oral imbalance in the future.

pH Neutralization

One of the most important factors in maintaining healthy teeth is pH. First, consider what pH means. It is a measure of acidity or alkalinity.

pH 0	Battery Acid
pH 1	Stomach Acid
pH 2	Lemon Juice, Vinegar
pH 3	Orange Juice, Soda, Some Dental Rinses
pH 4	Tomato Juice, Beer
pH 5	Black Coffee
pH 6	Saliva, Cow's Milk
pH 7	Pure Water
pH 8	Sea Water, pH-Neutralizing Dental Rinses
pH 9	Baking Soda
pH 10	Antacids
pH 11	Antacids, Dental Treatment Rinses
pH 12	Soapy Water

Figure 10. pH Scale

The lower the pH, the more acidic something is; and the higher the pH, the more alkaline something is. The pH scale goes from 1 to 14, 1 being the most acidic, 14 being the most alkaline, and 7 being neutral (like most water) (See Figure 10). A pH of 5.5 is an important pH level for teeth as the teeth begin to dissolve or demineralize at a pH in the mouth below 5.5. At a pH above 5.5, the teeth begin to remineralize (See Figure 11).

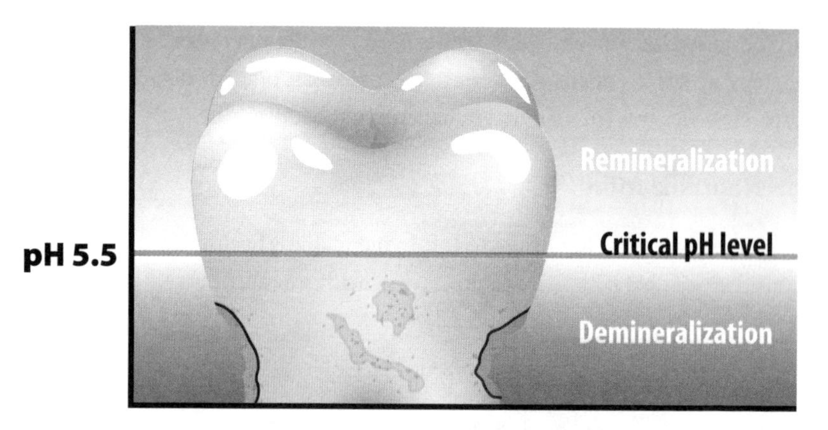

Figure 11. The results of being above and below the critical pH point of 5.5

Many oral microorganisms require a pH around neutrality for growth and are sensitive to extreme changes in acid or alkali. The pH of most surfaces in the mouth is regulated by saliva, which has a mean unstimulated pH of 6.75–7.25. Optimal pH values for healthy bacterial growth will be provided to the areas of the mouth bathed by saliva.[35] Shifts in the proportions of bacteria within the dental plaque from healthy to unhealthy occur following fluctuations in environmental pH.[35] When we eat, the pH in plaque can fall rapidly to below pH 5.0 through the production of acids (predominately lactic acid) as the bacteria metabolize (eat) the ingested nutrients.[35] Consuming acidic foods and drinks can likewise lower the pH within the mouth. Depending on the frequency (and the acidity) of food intake, the bacteria in plaque

> **Many oral microorganisms require a pH around neutrality for growth and are sensitive to extreme changes in acid or alkali.**

will be exposed to a variety of episodic challenges of low pH.[35] Many of the predominantly healthy bacteria within dental plaque (nonacid producers) can tolerate brief conditions of moderately low pH but are inhibited or killed by more frequent or prolonged exposures to acidic conditions.[35] If a patient's mouth experiences dramatic or long-lasting periods of low pH, this can result in the enhanced growth of, or colonization by, aciduric and acidogenic (cavity-causing) bacteria.[35]

Put simply, the equation looks like this:

Prolonged/intense low pH in the mouth = death of healthy bacteria/ overgrowth of cavity-causing bacteria = caries infection = CAVITIES.

Dental plaque that is kept at a pH of 7.0 or greater does not experience this shift in the bacterial species to aciduric and acidogenic (cavity-causing) bacteria even during exposure to sugar. If the pH in the mouth can be maintained at a neutral or alkaline pH, regardless of sugar, food, or acidic drink consumption, the healthy bacteria within the dental plaque biofilm will not die and the shift to cavity-causing bacteria will not occur.[36]

Many of the predominately healthy bacteria within dental plaque can tolerate brief conductions of moderately low pH but are inhibited or killed by more frequent or prolonged exposures to acidic conditions.[35] Dental plaque that is kept at a pH of 7.0 or greater does not experience this shift in the bacterial species to aciduric and acidogenic bacteria, even during exposure to sugar.

A healthy pH balance in the mouth can explain why many people—family members, coworkers, friends, etc.—can consume lots of sugary food and drink, seemingly take little care of their mouth, and yet do not have cavities. At the same time, many people who are extremely diligent about their diet and home care continue to get cavities because the bacteria in their biofilm are primarily cavity-causing bacteria. These people continue to be very susceptible to small changes in pH.

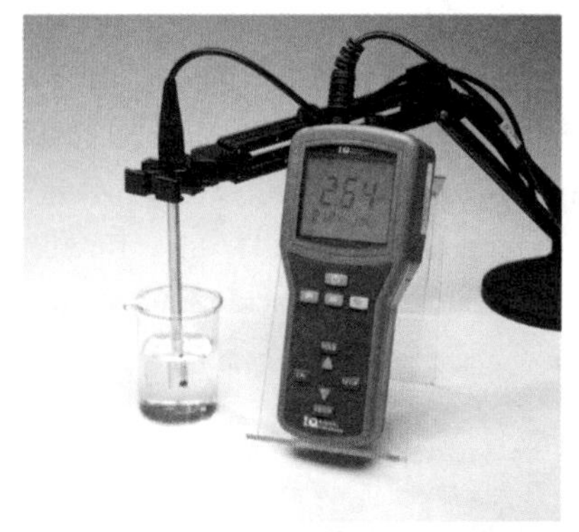

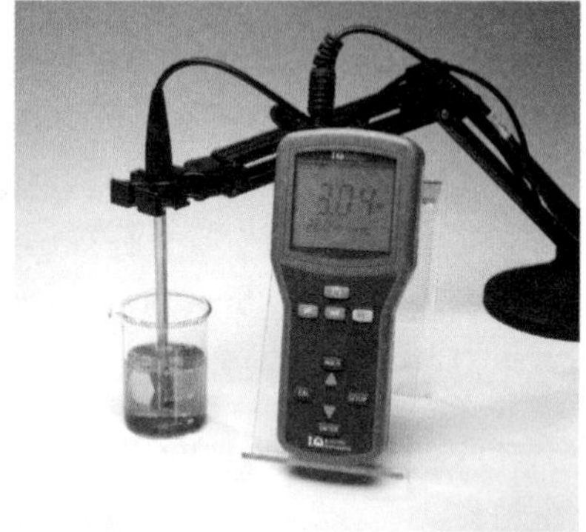

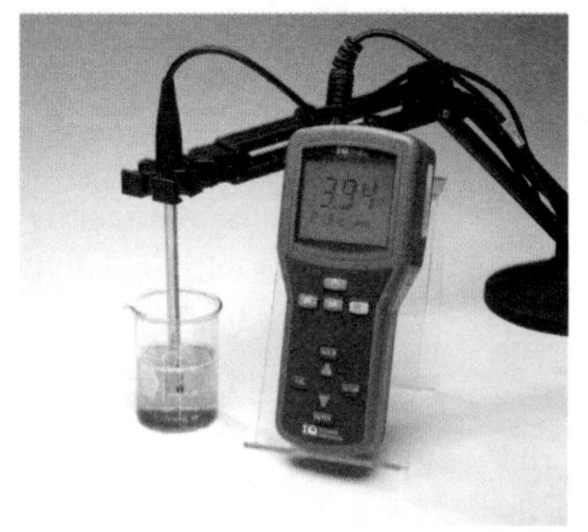

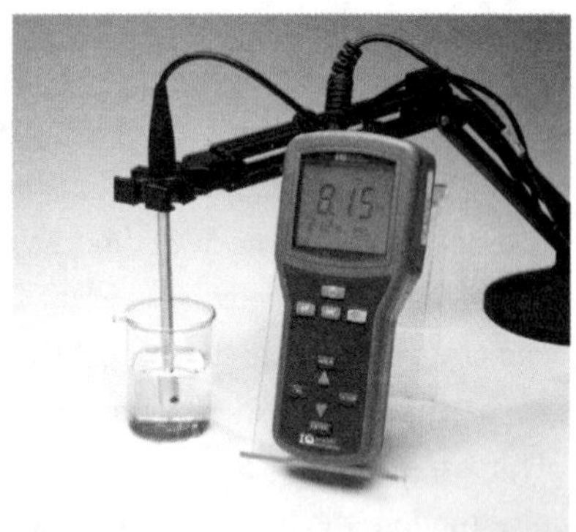

Figure 12. pH of 3 common over-the-counter oral rinses and one professional/prescription alkaline pH oral anticavity rinse (lowest to highest)

The good news is that this microbial shift from healthy bacteria to cavity-causing bacteria can be reversed using alkaline pH dental therapies (See Figure 12). The pH neutralization (alkaline) therapy can be used in a few different ways.

For those patients that are experiencing dental decay, alkaline dental products with pH ranges from 8 to 11 can be used daily to reverse the bacterial shift from cavity-causing bacteria to healthy bacteria. In addition, daily uses of a pH neutralizing oral spray, gel, or gum after meals, snacks, and drinks can quickly elevate acidic oral conditions caused by diet. This method of pH neutralization can shorten acid attacks caused by foods/sugars and keep the acid attack from dropping to intensely low pH levels.

Finally, for patients that have risk factors leading to a bacterial imbalance, targeted pH neutralization dental products used daily can greatly aid in preventing a bacterial shift in their oral biofilm. This is especially important for individuals with unmodifiable risk factors such as a restricted diet, saliva issues, prescription medications, and children at risk. It is preferable to prevent the bacterial shift from healthy to unhealthy (cavity-causing) than to reverse an acidic biofilm back to a healthy balance.

For those patients that are experiencing dental decay, alkaline dental products with pH ranges from 8 to 11 can be used daily to reverse the bacterial shift from cavity-causing bacteria to healthy bacteria.

In a clinical trial, conducted by the authors, examining the potential of pH neutralization as a caries treatment strategy, ten high caries risk adults were instructed to wear oral trays containing a gel with a pH of 9.0 for 8 hours at night for a period of 30 days. Mixed samples of their plaque were taken prior and after the 30-day period. The plaque samples from each individual were then checker-boarded using PCR and 16S gene sequencing DNA identification to identify the individual bacteria and the changes the bacterial species and concentration based on the neutralizing strategy. The results demonstrated an elimination of caries-causing bacteria like *Selenomonas*, slight reduction of *Streptococcus mutans/sobrinus*, *Lactobacillus* species, and a concurrent growth of healthy bacteria including *Prevotella*, *Campylobacter*, and *Veillonella* (See Figure 13). These limited results demonstrate that it is possible to reduce/shift the cariogenic microbes from the oral biofilm while replacing them with healthy organisms by regular maintenance of a neutral pH with a tray/gel system.

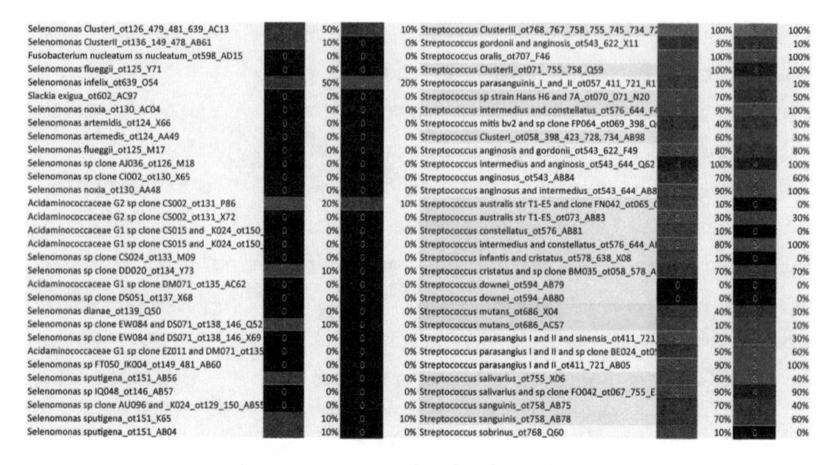

Selenomonas ClusterI_ot126_479_481_639_AC13	50%	10%	Streptococcus ClusterIII_ot768_767_758_755_745_734_7	100%	100%
Selenomonas ClusterII_ot136_149_478_AB61	10%	0%	Streptococcus gordonii and anginosis_ot543_622_X11	30%	10%
Fusobacterium nucleatum ss nucleatum_ot598_AD15	0%	0%	Streptococcus oralis_ot707_F46	100%	100%
Selenomonas flueggii_ot125_Y71	0%	0%	Streptococcus ClusterII_ot071_755_758_Q59	100%	100%
Selenomonas infelix_ot639_O54	50%	20%	Streptococcus parasanguinis_I_and_II_ot057_411_721_R1	10%	10%
Slackia exigua_ot602_AC97	0%	0%	Streptococcus sp strain Hans H6 and 7A_ot070_071_N20	70%	50%
Selenomonas noxia_ot130_AC04	0%	0%	Streptococcus intermedius and constellatus_ot576_644_F	90%	100%
Selenomonas artemidis_ot124_X66	0%	0%	Streptococcus mitis bv2 and sp clone FP064_ot069_398_Q	40%	30%
Selenomonas artemedis_ot124_AA49	0%	0%	Streptococcus ClusterI_ot058_398_423_728, 734_AB98	60%	30%
Selenomonas flueggii_ot125_M17	0%	0%	Streptococcus anginosis and gordonii_ot543_622_F49	80%	80%
Selenomonas sp clone AJ036_ot126_M18	0%	0%	Streptococcus intermedius and anginosis_ot543_644_Q62	100%	100%
Selenomonas sp clone CI002_ot130_X65	0%	0%	Streptococcus anginosus_ot543_AB84	70%	60%
Selenomonas noxia_ot130_AA48	0%	0%	Streptococcus anginosus and intermedius_ot543_644_AB8	90%	100%
Acidaminococcaceae G2 sp clone CS002_ot131_P86	20%	10%	Streptococcus australis str T1-E5 and clone FN042_ot065_	10%	0%
Acidaminococcaceae G2 sp clone CS002_ot131_X72	0%	0%	Streptococcus australis str T1-E5_ot073_AB83	30%	30%
Acidaminococcaceae G1 sp clone CS015 and _K024_ot150_	0%	0%	Streptococcus constellatus_ot576_AB81	10%	0%
Acidaminococcaceae G1 sp clone CS015 and _K024_ot150_	0%	0%	Streptococcus intermedius and constellatus_ot576_644_A	80%	100%
Selenomonas sp clone CS024_ot133_M09	0%	0%	Streptococcus infantis and cristatus_ot578_638_X08	10%	0%
Selenomonas sp clone DD020_ot134_Y73	10%	0%	Streptococcus cristatus and sp clone BM035_ot058_578_A	70%	70%
Acidaminococcaceae G1 sp clone DM071_ot135_AC62	0%	0%	Streptococcus downei_ot594_AB79	0%	0%
Selenomonas sp clone DS051_ot137_X68	0%	0%	Streptococcus downei_ot594_AB80	0%	0%
Selenomonas dianae_ot139_Q50	0%	0%	Streptococcus mutans_ot686_X04	40%	30%
Selenomonas sp clone EW084 and DS071_ot138_146_Q52	10%	0%	Streptococcus mutans_ot686_AC57	10%	10%
Selenomonas sp clone EW084 and DS071_ot138_146_X69	0%	0%	Streptococcus parasangius I and II and sinensis_ot411_721	20%	30%
Acidaminococcaceae G1 sp clone EZ011 and DM071_ot135	0%	0%	Streptococcus parasangius I and II and sp clone BE024_ot0	50%	60%
Selenomonas sp FT050_IK004_ot149_481_AB60	0%	0%	Streptococcus parasangius I and II_ot411_721_AB05	90%	100%
Selenomonas sputigena_ot151_AB56	10%	0%	Streptococcus salivarius_ot755_X06	60%	40%
Selenomonas sp IQ048_ot146_AB57	0%	0%	Streptococcus salivarius and sp clone FO042_ot067_755_E	90%	90%
Selenomonas sp clone AU096 and _K024_ot129_150_AB5	0%	0%	Streptococcus sanguinis_ot758_AB75	70%	40%
Selenomonas sputigena_ot151_K65	10%	10%	Streptococcus sanguinis_ot758_AB78	70%	60%
Selenomonas sputigena_ot151_AB04	10%	0%	Streptococcus sobrinus_ot768_Q60	10%	0%

Figure 13. DNA Checkerboard data

The method of pH neutralization is a safe and effective way of reversing the bacterial shift or preventing the bacterial shift toward cavity-causing bacteria and can be used for all age groups, including infants. Patients are encouraged to identify the pH of dental products they use in order to identify if the products are pH neutralizing. The ideal pH range for prevention is 8–9, and the ideal pH range for treatment of an unhealthy biofilm is 9–11.

Fluoride

Fluoride as a protective factor for tooth decay. There is abundant scientific evidence that demonstrates that fluoride strengthens the teeth, makes them less susceptible to acid attacks, and inhibits the production of acids by cavity-causing bacteria. The evidence for the anticaries efficacy of daily fluoride use is strong.[37] Tooth structure is primarily made up of the mineral hydroxyapatite, which demineralizes when the oral pH drops at or below 5.5. When the teeth are under an acid attack and fluoride is present during the remineralization process, hydroxyapatite particles combine with fluoride to form fluorapatite within the tooth structure. Fluorapatite is more resistant to acid attacks than hydroxyapatite as it does not begin to dissolve or demineralize until the pH drops to or below 4.5. In the window of pH 4.5–5.5 (See Figure 14), hydroxyapatite is dissolving in the enamel and fluorapatite is forming. As the pH cycles in a healthy balance in the mouth, in the presence of fluoride, this window of pH accounts for maturation of the enamel, making it stronger and more decay resistant (see See Figure 3).

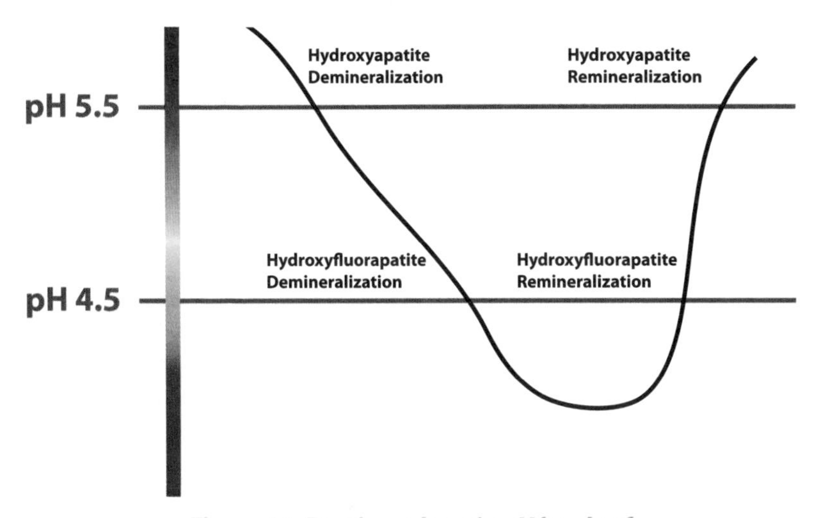

Figure 14. Demin and remin pH levels of hydroxyapatite and fluorapatite

Fluoride comes in many forms and concentrations. Neutral sodium fluoride can be used as a protective factor, and it comes in many concentrations and many different types of products. The most common are the following:

0.243% neutral sodium fluoride toothpaste/gel (over-the-counter/professional)

0.05% neutral sodium fluoride oral rinse (over-the-counter/professional)

1.1% neutral sodium fluoride toothpaste/gel (prescription)

5.0% neutral sodium fluoride varnish (prescription)

Based on your caries risk assessment, your dental professional will recommend proper products. For adults and children 6 years of age and older, any level of fluoride is considered safe and recommendations are made based on the patient's caries risk level. For children aged 2–5, the American Academy of Pediatric Dentistry recommends a pea-sized amount of 0.243% fluoride toothpaste/gel daily.[38] For children under age 2, due to the risk of fluorosis, other protective agents such as pH neutralization, xylitol, and nanoparticles of hydroxyapatite should be explored. Fluorosis results from higher-than-recommended levels/doses of fluoride exposure and appears as unsightly white spots or even brown spots on the teeth.

The greatest amount of therapeutic remineralization scientific evidence involves the use of fluoride. Numerous studies demonstrate the value of fluoride in the remineralization process.[39, 40, 41]

Xylitol

Xylitol has been recognized as an effective anticaries agent and also potentiates the effects of even small amounts of fluoride.[42, 43] Xylitol is a much less common anticaries agent than fluoride, and in the United States, the FDA only recognizes fluorides as "active ingredients" in anticaries products. One of the primary reasons xylitol is often limited to professional dental care and prescription grade products and not included in over-the-counter products is its cost. Xylitol is 5–6 times more expensive per kilogram than most common over-the-counter dental product sweeteners such as sorbitol. Also, in order to provide an effective "therapeutic dose" of xylitol, a dental care product should have a minimum concentration of at least 10%, while other sweeteners are used in much smaller concentrations.[44] While xylitol may be listed on many product labels, often patients and professionals must contact manufacturers or search their websites to determine how much xylitol is actually present in the product.

In order to provide an effective "therapeutic dose" of xylitol, a dental care product should have a minimum concentration of at least 10%.[44]

Xylitol is a five-carbon alcohol sugar. It is sweet in taste, similar to sugar (sucrose). Yet it works as an anticaries therapy agent in three ways. First, cariogenic bacteria cannot metabolize xylitol into acid, as they do many other carbohydrates and sweeteners, protecting the teeth from additional acid exposure. Second, because the bacteria cannot metabolize xylitol, it reduces their growth and a bacterial starvation effect occurs that over time can reduce total bacteria levels. Finally, because it is sweet tasting, it causes an increase in salivary flow to aid in the repair of damaged tooth enamel.

The dental product combination of sodium fluoride and xylitol can provide additional anticaries benefits of 12%.[44, 45]

Another proven benefit of xylitol is its synergistic therapy effect when combined with sodium fluoride. Xylitol can potentiate even very small levels of fluoride. The dental product combination of sodium fluoride and xylitol can provide additional anticaries benefits of 12%.[44, 45]

Xylitol is both noncariogenic in that it does not contribute to cavity formation and cariostatic because it prevents or reduces the incidence of new cavities. Xylitol actually reduces the amount of plaque and the number of bacteria in plaque. No other sugar substitute has been shown to function this way. Xylitol is safe for all age groups, and products specifically designed for children under the age of 2 are available. Xylitol can be found in oral rinses, sprays, toothpastes/gels, wipes, gums, and lollipops for children and adults.

Antibacterial

A broad-spectrum oxidizing antibacterial agent capable of penetrating a biofilm, such as sodium hypochlorite, should be considered as part of a treatment strategy.

Studies performed on the "killing" of biofilms have revealed some interesting results. While a "free floating" bacterial cell (planktonic) can be incredibly easy to kill, bacteria that have formed a biofilm can be incredibly resistant to antibacterials/antibiotics, etc.[46] Further observations using microscopy have revealed that the longer a bacterial biofilm population resides, the more ordered the biofilm structure becomes; and as the cells in the biofilm become more ordered and tightly packed, the biofilm becomes harder and harder to penetrate. Studies have shown that once bacteria cooperate and form a biofilm, packing tightly together, and establishing themselves, they further enhance their survival.[47] There are only three ways to remove or kill an established biofilm: complete mechanical debridement (which is impossible in the mouth), heat in excess of 400°F (which would destroy tooth structure), and a very strong oxidizing agent capable of penetrating a biofilm.[48] For this reason, a broad-spectrum oxidizing antibacterial agent capable of penetrating a biofilm, such as sodium hypochlorite, should be considered as part of a treatment strategy.

The medical management of dental caries has historically included fluoride in different delivery agents and antimicrobial or antibacterial therapy. Numerous antibacterial agents have been used, including ethyl alcohol, essential oils, chlorhexidine, and povidone-iodine. While ethyl alcohol can be an effective antibacterial agent, it has obvious issues and has also been linked to oral cancer.[49, 50, 51] Essential oils have been used for years as an antibacterial agent, but most commonly for the treatment of gum disease.

A standard antibacterial agent for dental caries has been chlorhexidine gluconate 0.12% rinse. There is a large body of evidence supporting the use of chlorhexidine as an antiplaque agent. The chlorhexidine molecule attaches to the bacterial cell wall and, after a prolonged period of contact, weakens the cell wall and eventually disrupts it. Chlorhexidine has a broad spectrum of action and has a significant effect against *Mutans streptococci* but has little effect on *Lactobacillus.* Clinicians recommending chlorhexidine rinse identified reduction of *MS* but also a coincident increase of *Lactobacillus* by bacterial culture of the saliva. Povidone-iodine 10%, or Betadine, has also been used as a dental caries antibacterial agent in limited applications.

Sodium hypochlorite 0.2% oral rinse is bactericidal to all bacteria on contact.

Povidone-iodine is a strong and broad-spectrum antibacterial agent that kills gram-positive and gram-negative bacteria, fungi, mycobacteria, viruses, and protozoans on contact. Povidone-iodine is effective against both *MS* and *Lactobacillus* in children when applied topically. Results from trials in adults demonstrated no anticaries effect. Problems associated with povidone-iodine as a rinse include taste and the limitation of using it only once a month because of the danger of iodine exposure, and it cannot be used by people with iodine or shellfish allergies. Aside from compliance issues, it also permanently stains clothing and countertops in the dental operatory.

Because dental caries is a biofilm disease, and biofilm diseases are best treated with a strong oxidizing agent, sodium hypochlorite has been introduced as an antibacterial agent. Sodium hypochlorite 0.2% oral rinse is bactericidal to all bacteria on contact. Limitations are alteration of taste and a recommendation to use it on patients aged 6 and older. As with all antibacterial agents, it should first be determined whether the patient has a bacterial biofilm load issue and would benefit from antibacterial therapy. The FDA considers oral rinse solutions with less than 0.3% concentration of sodium hypochlorite safe for daily use.

In another clinical trial, the authors examined the potential of 0.2% sodium hypochlorite rinse with a pH of 11 as an effective anticaries antibacterial agent. In the study, 5 high-caries-risk patients were instructed to rinse with the 0.2% sodium hypochlorite solution 2 times per day for a period of 30 days. Mixed samples of their plaque were taken prior and after the 30-day period. The plaque samples from each individual were then checker-boarded using PCR and 16S gene sequencing DNA identification to identify the individual bacteria and the changes in the bacterial species and concentration based on the antibacterial strategy. The plaque samples revealed an elimination of caries-causing bacteria like *Streptococcus mutans/sobrinus*, a reduction of *Lactobacillus*, and a concurrent growth of healthy bacteria including *Capnocytophaga, Prevotella, Campylobacter, Neisseria, Megasphaera, Veillonella, Eubacterium, Gemella, Granulicatella, Leptotrichia, Synergistes,* and *Actinomyces spp* (See Figure 15). These results demonstrate that it is possible to eliminate/reduce the cariogenic microbes from the oral biofilm while replacing them with healthy organisms by short-term therapy with a high pH antibacterial 0.2% sodium hypochlorite rinse strategy.

Gemella haemolysans_taxon626_K63	40%	60%
Gemella morbillorum_otn046_K64	60%	100%
Gemella morbillorum_ot046_AB09	20%	60%
Neisseria polysaccharia_gonhorreae_ot621_737_O76	0%	0%
Granulicatella adiacens_elegans_ot534_596_W81	20%	40%
Granulicatella adiacens_ot534_AB30	20%	40%
Granulicatella elegans_ot596_AB28	0%	0%
Granulicatella elegans_ot596_AB29	0%	0%
Lachnospiraceae MCE931_AO068_ot078_372_AB27	0%	0%
Lactobacillus ClusterI_ot568_716_749_W94	40%	40%
Lactobacillus acidophilus_not_oral_AC30	0%	0%
Lactobacillus acidophilus_not_oral_AC31	0%	0%
Lactobacillus delbrueckii_not_oral_AC28	0%	0%
Lactobacillus delbrueckii_not_oral_AC29	0%	0%
Lactobacillus fermentum_ot608_E51	40%	40%
Lactobacillus sp clone HT050_ot461_AD12	0%	0%
Lactobacillus gasseri and johnsonii_ot_615_819_V86	20%	0%
Ralstonia spp_not_oral_AD23	0%	0%
Lactobacillus salivarius_ot756_AB14	0%	0%
Leptotrichia wadeii_ot222_AD13	0%	0%
Lactobacillus sp HT070_ot461_AA66	0%	0%
Lactobacillus vaginalis_ot051_W93	0%	0%

Streptococcus ClusterIII_ot768_767_758_755_745_734_7	80%	100%
Streptococcus gordonii and anginosis_ot543_622_X11	20%	60%
Streptococcus oralis_ot707_F46	100%	100%
Streptococcus ClusterII_ot071_755_758_Q59	100%	100%
Streptococcus parasanguinis_I_and_II_ot057_411_721_R1	20%	0%
Streptococcus sp strain Hans H6 and 7A_ot070_071_N20	100%	80%
Streptococcus intermedius and constellatus_ot576_644_F	100%	100%
Streptococcus mitis bv2 and sp clone FP064_ot069_398_Q	20%	20%
Streptococcus ClusterI_ot058_398_423_728, 734_AB98	20%	0%
Streptococcus anginosis and gordonii_ot543_622_F49	100%	100%
Streptococcus intermedius and anginosis_ot543_644_Q62	100%	100%
Streptococcus anginosus_ot543_AB84	80%	100%
Streptococcus anginosus and intermedius_ot543_644_AB8	100%	100%
Streptococcus australis str T1-E5 and clone FN042_ot065_	0%	20%
Streptococcus australis str T1-E5_ot073_AB83	0%	0%
Streptococcus constellatus_ot576_AB81	0%	0%
Streptococcus intermedius and constellatus_ot576_644_A	100%	100%
Streptococcus infantis and cristatus_ot578_638_X08	0%	20%
Streptococcus cristatus and sp clone BM035_ot058_578_A	60%	40%
Streptococcus downei_ot594_AB79	0%	0%
Streptococcus downei_ot594_AB80	0%	0%
Streptococcus mutans_ot686_X04	20%	0%
Streptococcus mutans_ot686_AC57	0%	0%
Streptococcus parasangius I and II and sinensis_ot411_721	60%	40%
Streptococcus parasangius I and II and sp clone BE024_ot0	60%	80%
Streptococcus parasangius I and II_ot411_721_AB05	100%	100%
Streptococcus salivarius_ot755_X06	60%	100%
Streptococcus salivarius and sp clone FO042_ot067_755_E	100%	100%
Streptococcus sanguinis_ot758_AB75	40%	40%
Streptococcus sanguinis_ot758_AB78	60%	40%

Figure 15. DNA Checkerboard data

Sodium hypochlorite 0.2% oral rinse is also being prescribed for oral conditions other than caries. Clinicians have reported excellent results when prescribed for periodontal disease (biofilm imbalance below the gumline) as well as mouth ulcers (canker sores). Many patients who are undergoing dental treatment such as root canals, orthodontics, crown work or bridgework, and implants are provided 0.2% sodium hypochlorite oral rinse for home use to reduce the bioburden during restorative or cosmetic treatment plans.

Remineralization: Nanohydroxyapatite and Calcium Phosphate Ions

Dr. Philip Marsh first reported the biofilm nature of dental caries and prolonged periods of low pH, not sugar availability, as being responsible for the increase in acidic bacteria in the biofilm.[36] The shift in pH alters the components in the biofilm and leads to demineralization. In a healthy individual, following acid challenges, buffering agents and bacteria in the saliva and biofilm raise the pH and return it to a healthy pH, and then remineralization occurs.[36] This cycle repeats continuously throughout the day in our mouths.

In a healthy mouth, there is a balance between episodes of demineralization and remineralization with no resulting mineral loss from the teeth. This normal pH cycling in the mouth is considered healthy, where mineral is lost during periods of low pH and returns to the teeth during periods of higher pH. In dental caries, there is a loss of this balance with prolonged periods of low pH, favoring demineralization.

The body maintains healthy tooth mineral by replacing the lost hydroxyapatite and fluorapatite crystal particles as soon as the pH rises above critical remineralization pH.[52]

Remineralization occurs as a natural process within a healthy individual's mouth, and for this reason, some products are designed to mimic this process for the purpose of prevention and therapeutic strategies for dental caries. Remineralization is a complex process involving the condition of the existing tooth structure, the quantity and quality of saliva, the content and behavior of the bacteria biofilm, the presence of fluoride, and oral pH.

In order to understand remineralization, it is important to understand how tooth structure is designed and how the natural process works. Structurally, enamel is basically a crystal. When teeth form, they go through a process called amelogenesis, which is a process of crystal growth. In nature, crystals grow when in the right environment; nanoparticles of the crystal that are in a liquid or gas around a larger crystal move toward larger bodies of crystal and attach themselves. This is described as "oriented attachment"; the nano-sized crystals self-orient and attach themselves to larger crystals. Remineralization of the teeth works in the same way. The body maintains healthy tooth mineral by replacing the lost hydroxyapatite and fluorapatite crystal particles as soon as the pH rises above the critical remineralization pH.[52] For hydroxyapatite, this pH is 5.5, while for fluorapatite, the critical pH is 4.5. The basic building block of enamel is a crystallite about 20 nm in size.

While some have thought that calcium and phosphate are present in ionic forms in saliva, some of the mixed study results may be due to the fact that ionic forms of calcium phosphate generally do not occur in saliva unless salivary pH is influenced by outside sources.

Ionic Forms of Calcium Phosphate

Saliva is the solution around the tooth that allows for remineralization as it is supersaturated with brushite, octacalcium phosphate, tricalcium phosphate, fluorapatite, and hydroxyapatite nanoparticles—all forms of calcium phosphate.[53] Understanding this, and in an attempt to mimic natural remineralization, various forms of calcium phosphate ions have been included in some therapeutic strategies in addition to fluoride. Tricalcium phosphate, amorphous calcium phosphate, and CPP/ACP (casein phosphopeptide coated amorphous calcium phosphate) have all been added to different oral care products.[54, 55, 56] The scientific results in these topics are mixed; some conclude there is a lack of evidence or no benefit, while others demonstrate an improved result.[57, 58, 59, 60] While some have thought that calcium and phosphate are present in ionic forms in saliva, some of the mixed study results may be due to the fact that ionic forms of calcium phosphate generally do not occur in saliva unless salivary pH is influenced by outside sources, as the pH of resting saliva is about 6.75 and the pH of stimulated saliva is about 7.8, whereby the forms of calcium phosphate would only be available in nanocrystallite particle form. The biomimetic form of calcium phosphate is a 20 nm particle of hydroxyapatite.

Nanoparticles of Hydroxyapatite

Other non-ion forms of calcium phosphate materials have been used and studied as well. As hydroxyapatite and fluorapatite are present in greatest quantities in saliva and are the most bioavailable form for remineralization, they play the most significant role in remineralization. Hydroxyapatite and fluorapatite are present in supersaturated levels in saliva, and as the saliva flow increases during stimulated saliva flow, the degree of supersaturation also increases. Hydroxyapatite in nanoparticle crystallite form is also the most thermodynamically stable form

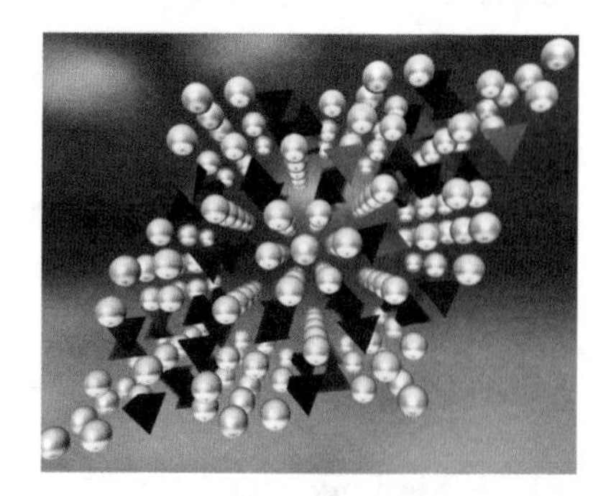

Hydroxyapatite crystal (conceptual image)

of calcium phosphate,[61] and studies examining nanoparticle hydroxyapatite as a biomimetic remineralization agent have been performed recently.[62,63,64] Studies demonstrate that nanoparticles in the 20 nm size (1/850th the width of a human hair) mimic the building blocks of natural enamel and are effective as an enamel repair material and anticaries agent.[65] Nanoparticle hydroxyapatite has also been demonstrated to restore luster to enamel damaged by bleaching agents.[63]

On the right in Figure 16 (scanning electron microscope) are images of extracted teeth used in a study on the remineralization potential of a nanohydroxyapatite gel used in conjunction with 1.1% neutral sodium fluoride, pH neutralization (pH of 9), and xylitol. The first image shows the natural tooth surface, the second shows artificial demineralization using 35% hydrogen peroxide, and the third shows the remineralization and attached particles of nanohydroxyapatite after the demineralized surface was brushed with the gel and placed in artificial saliva for 24 hours. Clinical trials are a challenge in examining remineralization, and it is difficult to duplicate in vivo (human) conditions during an in vitro (laboratory) study. Remineralization research is often limited to models with artificial lesions and saliva (as shown).[66, 67]

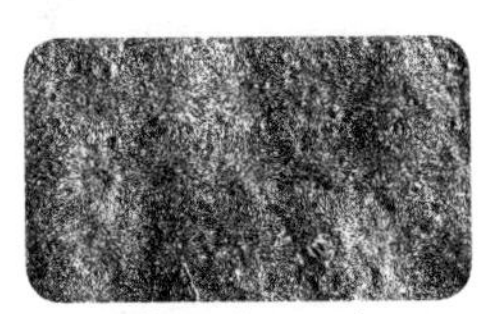

Normal enamel

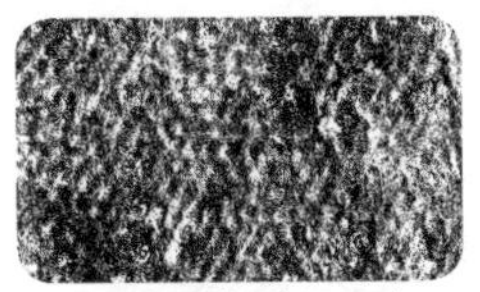

Demineralized enamel

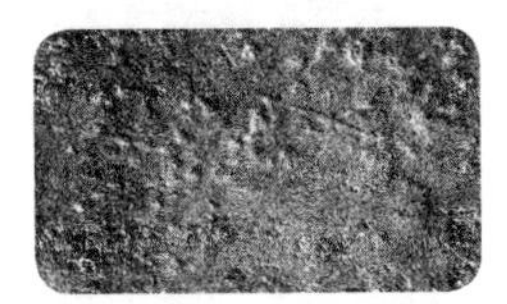

Remineralization after 24 hours

Figure 16. Remineralization of enamel with nanohydroxyapatite

Kois Center Research, a division of the Kois Center, LLC.

Numerous choices exist for patients looking to combat their risk factors with protective factors and weight their personal "caries balance" toward health. When considering a caries management therapy, always consult your dental professional and choose the most proactive therapy they recommend.

Step 5:

The Caries Risk Assessment Appointment

Historically, the dental "checkup" or hygiene appointment consisted of examining patients for signs/symptoms of oral diseases. Cavities caused by the caries infection, periodontal disease caused by a periodontal infection, accelerated wear of the teeth caused by a variety of oral environmental conditions such as bruxism (clenching), etc. Signs of disease are identified through a variety of methods, including x-rays, oral examination with an explorer or probe, and your dental practitioner's education and experience, while symptoms are generally reported by the patient. The historical dental appointment identified issues that presented after the damage has already been done. Caries risk assessment is a diagnostic method used to identify issues on the other "side of the equation" or before irreversible damage has occurred. This allows dental professionals and patients the opportunity to intervene with behavior modification and prescription/professional therapies.

Risk Factors

In most dental practices performing caries risk assessment, a patient's risk factors are identified in one of two ways. Either the patient is handed a risk assessment form prior to the appointment while in the reception area and asked to fill out the risk factor survey questions, or the dental hygienist/assistant interviews the patient regarding any risk factors they may have. However the information is gathered, the goal is simply to identify factors that may be placing the patient at risk for dental decay. Based on the present risk factors, the dental professional will use this information to help guide them when recommending prescription/professional product therapies targeted for specific risk issues or making restorative or cosmetic recommendations.

The goal is simply to identify risk factors that may be placing the patient at risk for dental decay.

Bacterial Biofilm Imbalance/Biofilm Challenge

If a biofilm challenge is found, the practitioner will make recommendations for antibacterial therapy.

In order to assess if a patient has a current bacterial imbalance on their teeth, any bacterial testing will be done prior to any x-rays, cleaning, or oral examination. The most common biofilm challenge test is the CariScreen Caries Susceptibility Test, which is a simple and painless swab sample test from the biofilm on the teeth (See "The Science of ATP Testing"). The CariScreen test provides a numerical result between 0 and 9999. A reading of 1500 or higher is indicative of a patient with a bacterial biofilm imbalance or more specifically a biofilm challenge.

Many patients assume that if they get a high reading, it means they have cavities, while others believe that if they have cavities, they are guaranteed a high CariScreen result. But this is not always the case. A high CariScreen test result simply means there is an abundance of bacteria and/or cavity-causing bacteria on the teeth. A low CariScreen test result means there is a low quantity of bacteria and/or cavity-causing bacteria on the teeth.

Just as a patient with low cholesterol can have a heart attack, or a patient who quit smoking 5 years ago can be diagnosed with lung cancer, the signs/symptoms of a disease, in this case cavitation in the teeth, do not always occur immediately after a risk factor or imbalance is detected. Like many diseases, there are multiple factors that contribute to the development of signs/symptoms. A patient who suffers a heart attack may not have high cholesterol, but they may have high blood pressure or inflammation in their arteries. Similarly, a patient with cavities may have a saliva issue, making them more susceptible to tooth decay even though their biofilm challenge is low. Or a patient with a high biofilm challenge and no current decay may simply not have any detectible cavities yet. The dental professional will use other caries risk assessment information to decide if the CariScreen test results or any other bacterial test results are of concern.

If a biofilm challenge is found, the practitioner will make recommendations for antibacterial therapy. If a biofilm challenge is not currently present, the practitioner will make recommendations based on other factors, and antibacterial therapy is not likely to provide a benefit for the patient.

Disease Indicators

> **Having signs/symptoms of the disease, cavities present, or a history of decay is the best predictor of cavities in the future.**

Disease indicators are signs of caries imbalance. Disease indicators include signs like new or progressing visible cavitations, new or progressing cavities detected by x-ray, new/active white spot lesions on the teeth, and a history (last 3 years) of decay. Having signs/symptoms of the disease, cavities present, or a history of decay is the best predictor of cavities in the future. Patients with a disease indicator found during their risk assessment have a 63.9–88% chance of new decay in the next 12 months without intervention.[23]

Because of the high likelihood of new decay if a disease indicator is found, practitioners make appropriate recommendations for reducing risk based on the patient's risk factors, biofilm challenge, and disease indicators. Patients with disease indicators should take their practitioners' therapy recommendations seriously. Not only do these patients have a very high likelihood of new decay in the next 12 months, but the current home care and therapy program they are using is obviously not providing enough protective factors to keep them in balance. Based on the patient's decay history and severity, long-term therapy may be necessary to get the patient back into balance and stop the decay process. Most patients respond fairly quickly, showing progress within 1–2 follow-up appointments if they adhere to daily recommendations. Some patients may require multiple follow-up visits and therapy modification to reduce their risk.

Step 6:

Caries Risk Assessment Patient Examples

Note: all patient examples have been taken from actual interviews, phone conversations, and e-mails with patients, practitioners, and CAMBRA experts. Patient names have been changed to protect privacy. Each category of examples includes a patient whereby their first caries risk assessment appointment placed them in that risk category. During their history, their risk may have increased or decreased based on their decisions and actions.

Low-Risk Patient (approximately 3% of the population)[68]

Mary

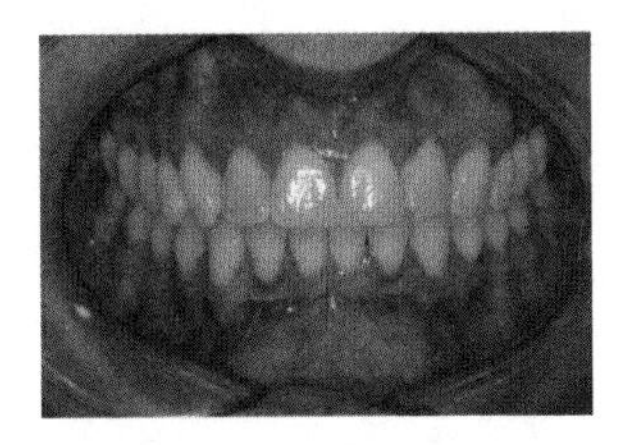

12/5/05: Mary is a 34-year-old stay-at-home mother with 2 children. She had a cavity 16 years ago when she was a teenager, and the experience dramatically changed her perspective on her oral care habits. Mary says that she brushes her teeth twice daily and flosses about once a week. She does admit to missing a brushing here and there due to her home life with young children. Most important, she does not have any risk factors. She is currently not taking any medications and does not snack or drink anything other than water between meals. Mary has been focused for the last few years on "getting back in shape" after her pregnancies and has kept a good "3 small meals a day" schedule. She does not have any plaque buildup or any other medical conditions. Her CariScreen test had a result of 226, showing that she did not have a biofilm challenge. She has not needed any dental work since her filling 16 years ago and, as a result, has no disease indicators. She is low risk for dental caries.

Mary's dental practitioner shared Mary's caries risk assessment results with her and encouraged her to continue with her current diet and home care program and to let her know if anything changes. To date, Mary has had no new cavities.

Moderate-Risk Patient (risk factors; approximately 23% of the population)[68]

Jeff

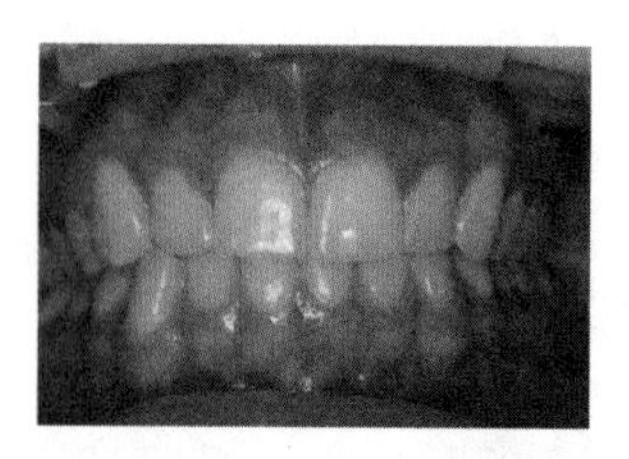

9/11/08: Jeff is a 26-year-old construction worker who often works long hours building homes. He has not had a single cavity in his entire life. He recently moved in with his fiancé and has plans to get married in 9 months. With his upcoming marriage, he wants to know about professional tooth whitening before his wedding. During his caries risk assessment, his dental practitioner found that he has a couple of risk factors for caries. With his long work hours, Jeff has been regularly drinking energy drinks throughout the day and does notice some plaque buildup every once in a while between brushings. His CariScreen score was 127, and he has no current cavities or other disease indicators. Due to his risk factors, he is moderate risk and has a 38.6% chance of new decay in the next 12 months.

Jeff's dental practitioner's concern regarding Jeff's caries risk was low, with his lack of cavities in the past and a couple of risk factors. But the practitioner suggested he cut back, if at all possible, on the energy drinks as they are highly acidic (pH 2.8–3.3) and contain sugar, but didn't see an issue performing the professional tooth whitening. Jeff said he didn't think stopping the energy drinks was an option right now with his heavy work hours and instead opted to use a pH neutralizing gum with xylitol after the energy drinks and meals. With his upcoming wedding, he didn't need an added dental expense or issue with his smile. He made a recall appointment as well as a separate whitening appointment. No history exists on Jeff past this appointment.

Elana

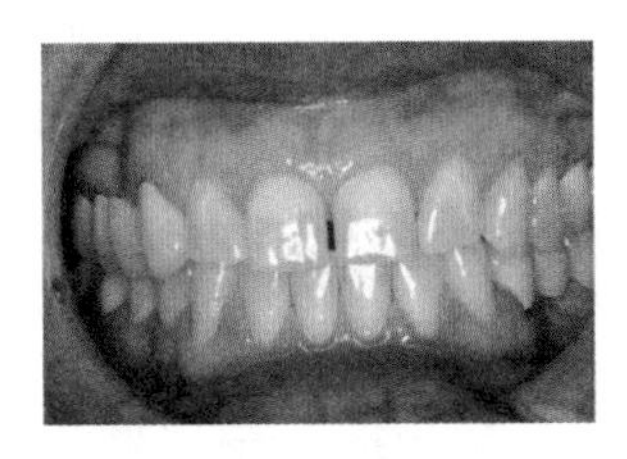

2/24/10: Elana is a 44-year-old high school teacher. She has not had any dental decay problems in the last 11 years. She had a low CariScreen score of 844 and no current disease indicators or cavities, but she had quite a few risk factors. She has been taking birth control and blood pressure medications for years and was recently diagnosed with moderate acid reflux. She has been taking 3 daily medications for the last 4 months and has felt like her mouth gets dry during her class lectures as well as at night. Because of the dry mouth, she has taken to drinking coffee and juices more often during the day. Not only did she notice some plaque buildup between brushings but the dental hygienist noted it as well. Elana reports that she brushes and flosses twice daily.

Statistically, Elana has a 38.6% chance of dental decay in the next 12 months, but the list of risk factors was a concern for her dental practitioner. Since Elana recently started some new medications that may be causing dry mouth and that these medications cannot be changed, the dental practitioner recommended that Elana use a 1.1% neutral sodium fluoride gel with xylitol, pH neutralization, and nanoparticles of hydroxyapatite along with a daily pH neutralizing spray with xylitol as needed for dry mouth. Elana said she was not interested in any therapy products at this time as they were not covered by her insurance.

9/15/10: Elana came back today for her 6-month checkup. Since her last appointment, she has increased her intake of juices and "other drinks" due to dry mouth, even though it causes her acid reflux to flare. Her CariScreen score was 1460, and she had two new cavities the dentist identified on her x-rays. The lack of saliva and frequent intake of acidic beverages were obviously making Elana more susceptible to infection. The dental practitioner made new therapy recommendations due to her increased caries risk and the presence of symptoms (cavities), but Elana again chose to decline as her fillings were covered by her dental insurance but the treatment products were not.

High-Risk Patient (risk factors and biofilm challenge; approximately 24% of the population)[68]

Roger

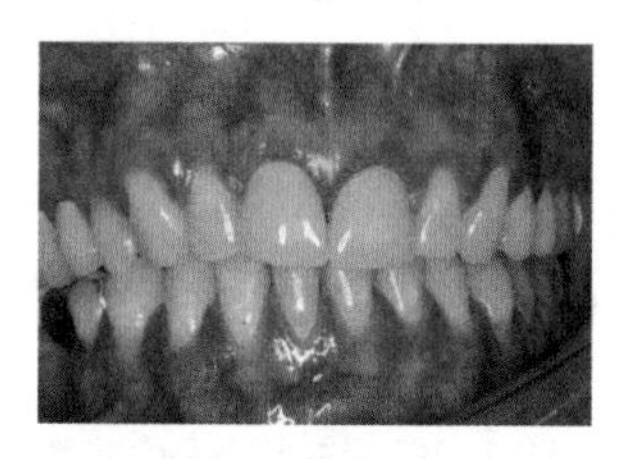

1/25/10: Roger is a 51-year-old police officer who has been seeing the same dentist for over 20 years. He hasn't had any decay in the last 9 years and has two risk factors. He takes a medication for high blood pressure and likes to drink 2 diet sodas a day while on the job and drinks 2–3 alcoholic drinks every night. His dentist had just recently started performing caries risk assessments and CariScreen testing. Roger's first CariScreen score was 4,125. Both he and his dentist were a little surprised at his biofilm challenge as he has had very good oral health throughout his lifetime. His dentist made some therapy recommendations, but as Roger has had good oral health and didn't feel his risk factors were "that bad," he opted not to make any therapy changes at this appointment.

8/6/10: Roger returned to his dentist for his next checkup, and none of his risk factors had changed. His CariScreen score at this appointment was 9889. At this point, the dental practitioner recommended a professional rinse and gel. The combination of the two products included antibacterial therapy with 0.2% sodium hypochlorite, pH neutralization, 1.1% neutral sodium fluoride, xylitol, and nanohydroxyapatite for remineralization. His dentist, who had known Roger for a long time, informed him that he had a 38%–69% chance of decay in the next 12 months, and he was concerned that at his age, something could change and he would start developing decay. Roger thanked his "doc" but again opted not to make any home care changes at this time.

6/10/11: Roger missed his regular 6-month appointment scheduled in February for unknown reasons. At this checkup, he did not share any new risk factors and marked his risk assessment form with the same two risk factors as before. His CariScreen score was 8227, and he had 4 new cavities. His dentist asked him if there had been any major changes in his life or any health concerns since his last appointment. Roger shared that he had hurt his back around Thanksgiving of the prior year and had been on pain and muscle relaxant medication for 3½ months while his back healed. But he wasn't taking the medications anymore. During that time, Roger had experienced minor dry mouth but hadn't changed any of his other eating or drinking habits because of it. His dentist recommended he get his cavities filled and again recommended a home care change with the combination of the two products with antibacterial therapy, pH neutralization, 1.1% neutral sodium fluoride, xylitol, and nanohydroxyapatite for remineralization. Roger decided it was time to follow his dentist's advice and began the therapy regimen.

12/15/11: Roger returned for his 6-month checkup and informed his dentist he had been using the therapy products 2 times daily for the last 6 months as he had recommended. The two risk factors of antihypertensive medication and drinks other than water more than 2 times daily were present. His CariScreen score was still elevated at 3460, but he had no new cavities. His dentist also noted that his gums looked healthier. Roger is still using the prescribed home care regimen daily.

Jennifer

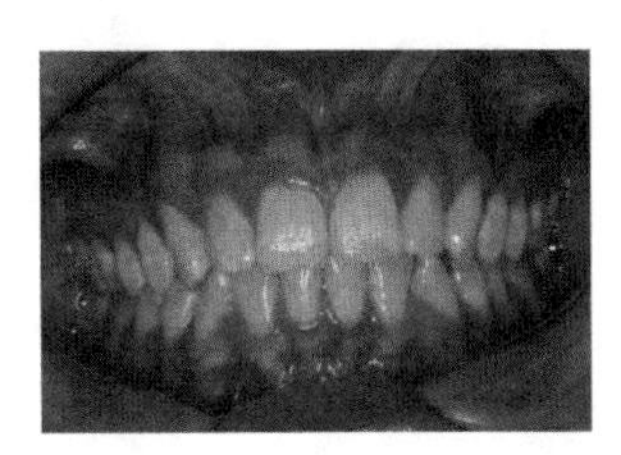

5/16/11: Jennifer is an active 32-year-old mother of 2 and works as a paralegal. She has not had any issues with dental decay since she was a child. When she was 5 years old, she had three fillings in her primary teeth but has had no issues since. She ran track in high school and has always enjoyed distance running. She has had the same dentist for 12 years. On her first caries risk assessment, she had two risk factors, frequent snacking and drinks other than water more than 2 times daily. She had a CariScreen score of 5870 but did not have any cavities at this appointment.

Jennifer's dental professional shared with her how the snacking and drinks increased her risk for dental decay and that her high CariScreen score was a concern. Jennifer responded that she was preparing for her first half marathon, and part of the preparation included a frequent intake of protein and carbohydrates. Also while running, she focused on maintaining her hydration and energy level by consuming sports drinks and small packets of honey with caffeine in them. As she was dedicated to her sport and felt the diet and drinks were necessary, she was not willing to make changes to her risk factors. She was concerned about her biofilm challenge and, as an individual who focused on making healthy choices, felt adding the prescription/professional home care products to her dental home care program was the right choice for her at this time. She decided to follow her dental professional's recommendation and start using an antibacterial rinse with 0.2% sodium hypochlorite, fluoride, xylitol, and pH neutralization, followed by a toothpaste/gel with 1.1% neutral sodium fluoride, xylitol, pH neutralization, and nanoparticles of hydroxyapatite 2 times daily. She scheduled a follow-up appointment in 3 months to reassess how her therapy choices were working.

8/21/11: Jennifer returned for her reassessment appointment, and none of her risk factors had changed. She had finished her first half marathon over the summer and was training for a full 26.2-mile marathon. Her CariScreen score at this appointment was 7762. Initially, she thought that maybe the therapy hadn't been working. But upon further discussion, she shared that her meals and drinks intake had increased with her workout increase. Her dental professional also shared that unless the risk factors were decreased, it might take multiple therapy cycles to lower her biofilm challenge. Second, if Jennifer added any additional risk factors while her biofilm challenge was so high, decay might develop. Jennifer chose to continue with the therapy and began another 3-month cycle.

11/17/11: Jennifer returned for her 6-month recare appointment. Nothing had changed with regard to her risk factors and lifestyle. Her CariScreen score was 4736, and she had no new decay. The dental professional noted that her gums did appear healthier than her last recare appointment, and Jennifer decided to continue with another cycle of therapy products.

2/20/12: Jennifer came in for a caries reassessment appointment. She had continued running, eating, and drinking at elevated levels, including 5 small meals per day with one snack and 10–12 energy drinks and 3–4 energy packets per week while working out. Her CariScreen score was 1544, and while her score was still elevated (above 1500), her dental professional was glad to see her moving in the right direction and was less concerned about her caries risk. Jennifer's dental professional suggested that Jennifer switch to a slightly different rinse that did not contain an antibacterial ingredient but still contained pH neutralization, xylitol, and fluoride and continue the toothpaste/gel with 1.1% neutral sodium fluoride, xylitol, pH neutralization, and nanoparticles of hydroxyapatite 2 times daily. As Jennifer's lifestyle will continue to include risk factors, her dental professional informed her that in order to avoid decay, Jennifer would need to continue using additional protective factor pH neutralizing products with xylitol, fluoride, and remineralization agents for as long as her risk factors were present.

High-Risk Patient (risk factors and disease indicators [decay] present, low biofilm challenge, approximately 19% of the population)[68]

Amelia

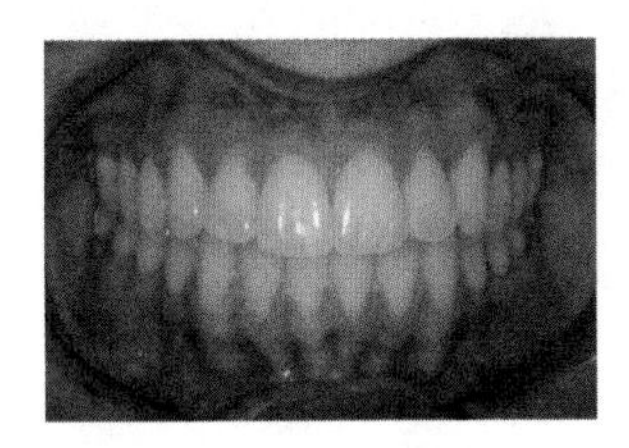

1/21/11: Amelia is a 23-year-old female with little dental history. She has not seen her dentist in 3 years and, 3 years ago, was a new patient who had no cavities or problems at all. She has recently started a job that includes dental insurance and has scheduled a cleaning appointment. During her caries risk assessment, she only self-reported that she sipped drinks other than water more than 2 times daily, but only on healthy drinks like tea and juice. Her CariScreen score was 622, but she had 4 new cavities visible on her x-rays; and during her examination, the dental professional noted it appeared Amelia had not been regular with her home care. Her dental professional was shocked her CariScreen score was so low. Amelia did not seem very forthcoming with information on her risk factors and said she only wanted what her dental insurance would cover. Her dental professional shared that they were there to help her in any way they could and that their goal was to help her improve her oral health. Amelia chose to decline any professional/prescription therapy products and scheduled the fillings covered by her dental insurance.

2/6/11: Amelia returned for her fillings, and her dentist noted her saliva did not seem normal and was thick and sticky. The dentist inquired regarding her risk factors and CariScreen score and asked her if there was anything else going on in her life that could be affecting her diet or if she felt like she had a dry mouth. Amelia again chose not to share any risk factor information with her dentist.

7/19/11: Amelia returned for her 6-month recall visit, and she did not self-report any other risk factors other than her frequent daily drinks of tea and juice. Her CariScreen score was 536, and she had one new cavity that needed restoration, a couple small new lesions forming, and as some recurrent decay around one of her previous fillings. Her hygienist inquired as to why Amelia liked to have liquids to drink so frequently. Amelia informed her hygienist that she kept them close because she felt like her mouth was dry sometimes. At this point, her hygienist pulled out Amelia's caries risk assessment form and went through the risk factor list, covering each question thoroughly but without judgment, knowing something was missing. Amelia was initially resistant, but as the hygienist continued to ask open-ended questions, Amelia began to share and the dental team discovered that Amelia was actually on 4 different medications for depression, anxiety, and back pain that she took daily. Amelia was initially resistant to share her medications as she didn't feel they were important to her dentist and felt embarrassed about the medications she was taking. During a visit to a local medical clinic a year ago, she had been treated like a "drug seeker" and was tired of feeling judged. She was working hard and was taking care of her mother and little brother and felt that few medical professionals took her seriously. It took her dental team time to build enough trust for her to share some risk factors that were making her more susceptible to dental decay. After understanding the underlying cause of her susceptibility and the options she had, Amelia had an in-office fluoride varnish and chose to begin using a professional rinse and toothpaste/gel with pH neutralization, xylitol, fluoride, and nanoparticles of hydroxyapatite at home.

10/12/11: Amelia returned for a 3-month recall check to assess how her therapy was working. She was still taking the 4 different medications and experiencing dry mouth. She was also still frequently sipping tea and juice. Thankfully, her early lesions identified at the previous visit were showing signs of remineralization and all of her restorations looked great. Due to her low saliva flow, it was important that she continue with a maintenance program of pH neutralization, xylitol, fluoride, and nanoparticles of hydroxyapatite; and Amelia chose to stick with using the professional rinse and toothpaste/gel with pH neutralization, xylitol, fluoride, and nanoparticles of hydroxyapatite daily.

To date, Amelia has shown no new decay.

Jerome

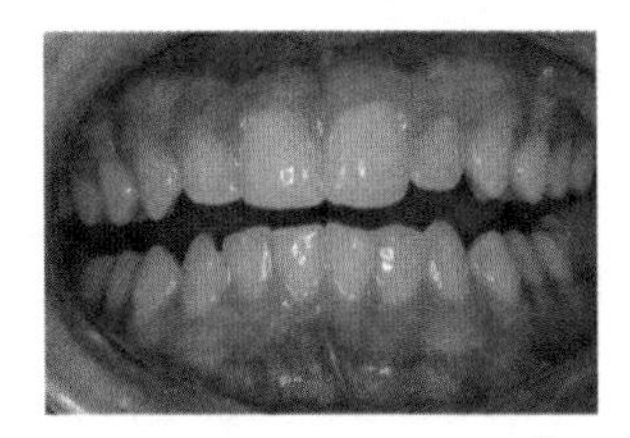

7/12/11: Jerome is a 17-year-old high school athlete. He has had numerous problems with decay in the last 3 years. His first caries risk assessment revealed that he only had one risk factor: drinking liquids other than water more than 2 times daily. He had excellent oral hygiene habits and was brushing with an electric toothbrush twice daily as well as flossing daily. He had a CariScreen score of 989 and 4 new cavities as well as some other early lesions the dentist wanted to keep an eye on. He shared that he very regularly consumed diet sodas as well as diet sports drinks due to his daily sports routine and had basically stopped drinking anything else during the day. His dentist explained how both diet sodas and sports drinks were extremely acidic (pH 2.5–3.3). The regular bathing of Jerome's teeth in acid and some sugars (in the diet sports drink) were causing even the low level of bacteria on his teeth to cause cavities. He said he would try to limit the diet soda and drink more water during his physical activities. He chose to be conservative with his home care program and replaced his toothpaste with the one the dentist recommended that had 1.1% neutral sodium fluoride, pH neutralization, xylitol, and nanoparticles of hydroxyapatite for remineralization.

2/2/12: Jerome returned for a 6-month checkup, and his caries risk assessment revealed the same risk factor of liquids other than water more than 2 times daily. His CariScreen score was 1027, and two of the areas the dentist had chosen to watch previously now had decay that needed restoration. But Jerome had two other spots that appeared to have partially remineralized. He shared that he had cut out most of the diet soda but was still consuming 4–5 diet sports drinks on a daily basis. He had a couple of choices: He could choose to keep his same home care program and sports drink consumption and continue getting cavities; although he had slightly less this time, he was still showing signs of the disease. He could choose to increase his home care regimen, which included both prescription toothpaste/gel and a professional oral rinse with pH neutralization, fluoride, xylitol, and nanoparticles of hydroxyapatite for remineralization, or decrease his sports drink consumption. He chose to up his home care program and said he would try to cut back on the sports drinks. He and his parents were tired of all the new cavities, and he really wanted to look into orthodontics and whitening. But his parents said that they weren't going to pay for any cosmetic dental work until he stopped getting cavities, and his dentist agreed. Adding orthodontic brackets to his teeth would just increase his risk at this point. Jerome's dentist wanted him to come back in 3 months when his home care kit was gone and reassess if the new therapy program was enough to get him under control.

5/22/12: Jerome came back in for his 3-month reassessment, and his CariScreen score was 416. His dentist noticed multiple areas of remineralization on his teeth, and he had no new cavities. Jerome explained that he had been extremely vigilant with his home care program of rinsing and then brushing but had actually increased his diet sports drink consumption. He also explained that he had taken the dental hygienist's advice, and whenever he drank the sports drinks during his athletic events, he drank them quickly and then did a quick rinse and spit with regular water to get the liquid off his teeth. This method had reduced the amount of acidic exposure to his teeth. Combined with the increase in protective factors he had, for the moment, found a balance. His dentist said he should keep up his program, and they would revisit his desire for orthodontics and whitening in 6 months if his balance was maintained.

High / Extreme-Risk Patient (risk factors and disease indicators [decay] present, high biofilm challenge; approximately 30% of the population)[68]

Jack

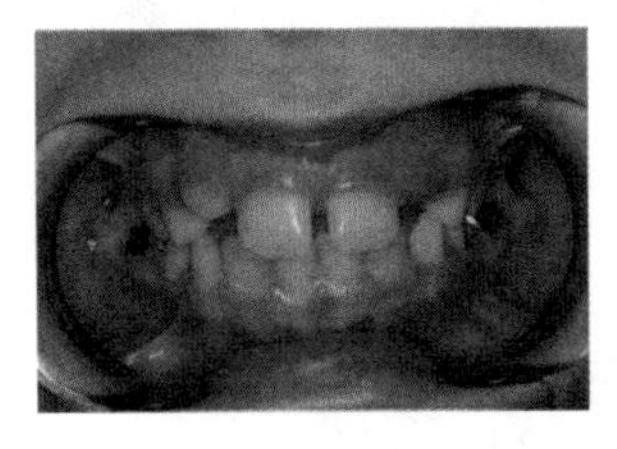

11/10/10: Jack is a 7-year-old boy with a recent history of decay. His parents had been taking him every 6 months for his dental checkups and cleanings, and they were frustrated with the decay at his last few appointments. Jack's only risk factor reported was plaque buildup between brushings, and his parents said they participated in Jack's daily home care and monitored his food and drink intake fairly closely. Jack had had 2–3 new cavities every year in the last couple of years and "freaks out a bit" because he was scared every time he came to the dental office. Everyone in the dental office remembers Jack, and he and his family were extremely frustrated with his continuous dental decay. His dentist thought of Jack when she implemented a new caries risk assessment and testing program and wasn't surprised that Jack's first CariScreen score was 8894 and at this appointment had 5 new cavities. After some conversation with Jack's mother, the dentist discovered that although the mother had not marked it on the CRA form, Jack also had other risk factors such as frequent snacking as well as drinks other than water more than 2 times daily. The mother had not shared that information on the CRA form as she didn't think the fruit, vegetables, cheese, raisins, milk, apple/pomegranate juice, and other healthy snacks Jack was snacking on daily "really counted." She thought they were only asking about soda and candy consumption. Jack's dentist shared how the pH in Jack's mouth was basically always low due to the frequency of his eating, drinking, and snacking; and this had caused the bacteria in Jack's mouth to become out of balance. The mother did not want to take away Jack's snacks as she felt it would be too much of a change in his daily routine and chose to add a 0.2% sodium hypochlorite antibacterial rinse with xylitol, pH neutralization, and fluoride to his daily home care program. She did not opt for the recommended 1.1% neutral sodium fluoride gel with pH neutralization, xylitol, and nanoparticles of hydroxyapatite for remineralization because she said Jack really liked using his "sparkly blue movie car" toothpaste. The dentist informed the mother that the antibacterial rinse did not taste great and that she would have to work with Jack to make sure he was using it twice a day for the next 6 months.

6/22/11: Jack came in for his 6-month checkup, and his CRA form revealed a new risk factor. Not only did Jack still have the other three risk factors of plaque buildup between brushings, frequent snacking, and drinks other than water more than 2 times daily; but he was now on a daily allergy medication that might be causing some dry mouth as he had increased his juice consumption. His CariScreen score was 9999, and he had 3 new cavities. His mother was frustrated and had informed Jack's hygienist that the antibacterial rinse wasn't working. After a thorough conversation with the mother, Jack's dentist discovered that Jack was only using the rinse a couple of times a week and the mom admitted she simply didn't like trying to get him to use it because, like his allergy medication, he "didn't like it." The dentist informed the mother that if they wanted to get his decay under control, something was going to have to change; they should choose one major change to Jack's routine and stick with it for 6 months and then reassess if more changes were necessary. The mother really did not want to change his eating/snacking routine as it really helped keep Jack busy, especially when his medication made him hyper. The mother chose to move forward with a professional home care kit for high/extreme-risk patients that covered all of the bases of antibacterial (0.2% sodium hypochlorite), fluoride, xylitol, pH neutralization, and nanohydroxyapatite for remineralization.

12/12/11: Jack returned for another 6-month checkup, and his mother only reported two risk factors, frequent snacking and drinks other than water more than 2 times daily. She said his plaque between brushing wasn't happening anymore and he was off the allergy medication during the winter. His CariScreen score was 2247, and he only had one very small cavity that had formed around an old filling. Both he and his mother had been using the professional products that had been recommended (she was also high/extreme risk), and Jack was excited to be using the "same toothpaste as his mom because he was a man now." The mother also mentioned that her mouth felt much cleaner and her gums had stopped bleeding when she flossed. She chose to continue using the professional home care kit (for both her and Jack) rather than changing Jack's eating and drinking habits.

6/2/12: Jack had no new cavities at this checkup! His CariScreen score was 2420, and his mother kept working diligently with him on his home care rather than changing his diet. They continue to use the professional home care kit with antibacterial (0.2% sodium hypochlorite), fluoride, xylitol, pH neutralization, and nanohydroxyapatite for remineralization every 3 months for Jack until everything is in balance or they choose to make dietary changes.

Sheila

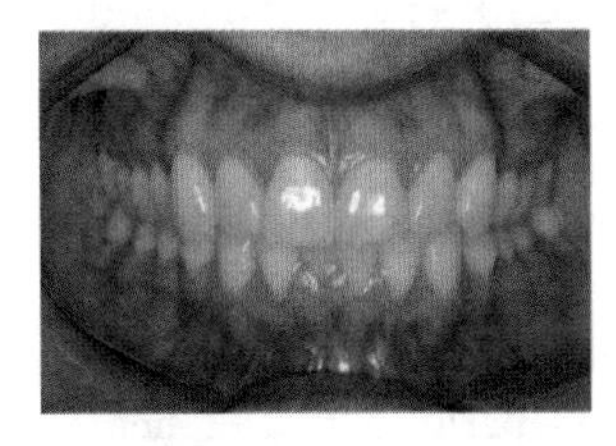

7/12/11: Sheila is a 36-year-old hygienist who works in a large group dental practice. While training on the CariScreen Caries Susceptibility Test, which was new technology for their practice, she and one of her fellow hygienists performed practice tests on each other. While Sheila had a few cavities as a child, she had not had any decay for many years and was "fanatical" about her oral hygiene. She was flabbergasted when her test showed a result of 9232. She shared that she did have a couple of risk factors in that she did take a couple of medications and was on a diet that required 5 small meals a day and one snack. Her CariScreen trainer shared with her that the CariScreen doesn't know if you are a hygienist, a dentist, or a bank robber. It provides an unbiased reading on the amount of biofilm ATP collected from the teeth. Sheila decided that she wanted to have the dentist check her out as it had been 10 months since her last x-rays. Upon inspection and x-ray, her dentist found two very early lesions forming between her back teeth. The dentist shared that she took a "hard look" at the x-rays knowing what Shelia's biofilm challenge was and identified the early decay. But the lesions were not big enough to necessitate fillings at this time, and Sheila could try remineralization therapy first. As Sheila processed the information, she began to connect the dots and realized that starting that extra medication 6 months ago, combined with the new diet 4 months ago, might have had an effect on her risk for decay, but she had made no changes to her oral care routine. She decided to attack the issue head-on and started professional home care kit with antibacterial (0.2% sodium hypochlorite), fluoride, xylitol, pH neutralization, and nanohydroxyapatite for remineralization that day.

7/30/11: Sheila called to inform her trainer that she had been using the professional home care kit for a couple weeks and decided to have another CariScreen test. The CariSceen reading was 9987, and she was concerned that the products weren't working, although her teeth did feel cleaner. Her trainer shared that it might be too early to see results and that she needed to finish the kit and retest at 3 months. Sheila decided to keep with it.

10/16/11: Sheila had another CariScreen test done by one of her coworkers, and her score was 4389. She was glad to see it had come down. Her dentist wasn't able to perform another x-ray at this time to check on the status of the early decay that was identified, so they decided to wait until 6 months. Sheila decided to keep up the professional home care kit and added an oral spray with pH neutralization and xylitol during the day after her meals and snack to elevate the pH in her mouth after eating her 5 daily meals and snack. She also shared that she had lost 7 pounds on her new diet.

2/4/12: Sheila had another CariScreen and x-rays performed. Her dentist said that her early decay appeared to have remineralized, and Sheila was very happy about that. But what she was most excited about was that her CariScreen score was 1610. Although it was a bit above the threshold, she was confident that a good home regimen with a professional home care kit including pH neutralization, xylitol, fluoride, and nanoparticles of hydroxyapatite and using the mouth spray after meals and snacks could keep her biofilm challenge down. She also said that she was planning a full "cosmetic dental makeover" for this summer. Being a hygienist, she had always wanted "perfect teeth." But she had always been worried about investing in a makeover for her teeth as she had seen people both with decay and without decay have full cosmetic makeovers and come back a year later with a new decay and their beautiful dental work breaking down. But now she was much more confident she could keep her risk in check, and after a divorce and losing 13 pounds, she was going to go for it!

Joyce

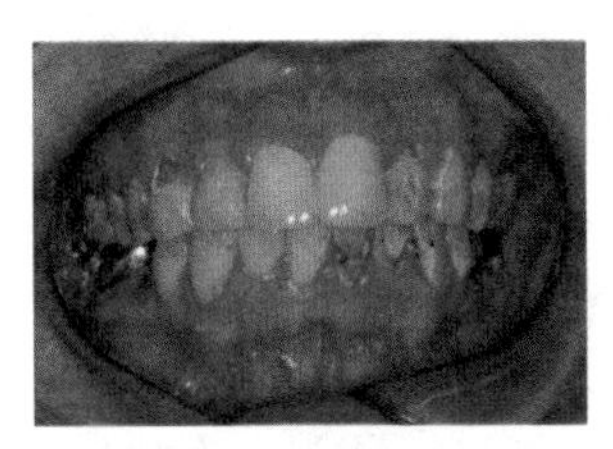

1/13/10: Joyce is a 38-year-old advertising client manager for a local radio station. She had had a lifelong battle with dental decay that had seriously impacted her life. She came in as a new patient to the dental practice because she heard from a friend that they could "cure" her dental decay problems. Her previous dentist was recommending she consider dentures, but she didn't want to lose all her teeth. She shared with her dental practitioner that she believes the poor esthetics of her teeth was one of the reasons her husband left her and that she believes her job might be in jeopardy due to her continued challenge of obtaining clients for the radio station. Her job is dependent on obtaining new advertising clients, and every time she would meet potential new clients face-to-face, they would seem to shy away the second she smiled. So she had simply stopped smiling altogether.

Joyce had always dreamed of having a "perfect Hollywood" smile, but she had given up on dentistry because she had always had decay and kept getting new decay every time she had her teeth restored. She had tried every dental product she could find at the supermarket and online, even some toothpaste from Japan, but nothing had helped.

Joyce's caries risk assessment had three risk factors: frequent snacking, drinks other than water more than 2 times daily, and two or three medications daily. She loves to drink coffee and other caffeinated drinks like tea (she takes all her clients and potential clients to the local coffee shop) and had been taking oral contraceptives, a daily over-the-counter acid reflux medication, and ibuprofen for dental pain. Her CariScreen score was 9268, demonstrating a biofilm challenge, and she had obvious extensive active decay.

Joyce wanted to know what her options were and asked her new dentist if she could be "cured" and have a "Hollywood smile," or if dentures really were her only option. Her dentist explained that due to her high caries risk, placing esthetic restorations like crowns, bridges, and veneers was not a viable option at this time as the likelihood of failure was very high. But Joyce did have other options than dentures. The dentist shared that she was going to have one tooth removed as it was nonrestorable and indicated for extraction. She had the option of having all of her necessary fillings done with a provisional "GIC" (glass ionomer cement) material that can act as a fluoride reservoir on her teeth while they worked together to design a plan to correct her oral biofilm imbalance with professional/prescription therapies and diet modification.

Joyce was overjoyed that she had an option other than dentures but didn't feel like she was ready to give up her coffee, and couldn't change her necessary medications. Her dentist suggested she use a medicated oral rinse and tooth gel twice daily with an antibacterial (0.2% sodium hypochlorite), 1.1% neutral sodium fluoride, xylitol, pH neutralization, and nanoparticles of hydroxyapatite for remineralization support. The dentist also suggested they make Joyce some "whitening trays" and that she wear the pH neutralizing gel with xylitol, nanoparticles of hydroxyapatite, and 1.1% neutral sodium fluoride in the trays at night while she slept. Joyce chose to move forward with the dentist's recommendations for the extraction, GIC provisional restorations, and professional/prescription therapy products at home. She wanted to know at what point she would be able to move forward with cosmetic restorations and have a bright white smile. The dentist shared that, due to her condition and high risk, he wouldn't feel comfortable placing those restorations until Joyce had multiple healthy appointments with no new decay (18–24 months healthy). Joyce said she was on a mission and agreed to the treatment plan.

6/22/10: Joyce returned for a 6-month cleaning appointment after having all of her restorations done with the provisional "GIC" material, the single tooth extracted, and using the recommended therapy products for 6 months at home. Her CariScreen score was 8338, and she still had the three risk factors of frequent snacking, drinks other than water more than 2 times daily, and daily medications (oral contraceptive and acid reflux medication). But she shared that she was not taking ibuprofen for dental pain any longer. Joyce had been diligent about her home care routine. She was rinsing twice daily with a rinse that contained an antibacterial (0.2% sodium hypochlorite), xylitol, pH neutralization (pH 11), and 0.05% fluoride. She then followed the rinse twice daily with a tooth gel that contained 1.1% neutral sodium fluoride, xylitol, pH neutralization (pH 9), and nanoparticles of hydroxyapatite. She was also wearing whitening trays with the same tooth gel in it at night. Her hygienist noted that her gums were much healthier, and Joyce said that they no longer bled when she flossed. Her dentist said that she had one small area of recurrent decay around a filling but multiple sites of remineralization and no new cavities. The dentist had to practically restrain Joyce from dancing in the operatory. Joyce was so happy, and after 20 minutes of joyful tears and hugs for the dental team, Joyce chose to have her recurrent decay repaired and continue with her home care program.

9/20/10: Joyce came in today for a check-up appointment, and nothing had changed with regard to her risk factors or home care program. Joyce continued to rinse and brush twice daily with the recommended products and wear the trays with gel in it at night. She did ask the dentist if her trays could be repaired as they had cracked in a few places from use. Her CariScreen score at this appointment was 3675, and her hygienist was so excited to see it coming down. She still had the three risk factors of frequent snacking, drinks other than water more than 2 times daily, and daily medications (oral contraceptive and acid reflux medication). The dentist did a thorough examination and found no new or recurrent decay. Joyce was overjoyed and wanted to know if they could plan the cosmetic restorations she wanted. The dentist said that she was well on her way, and if she could keep her mouth in balance for another 12–18 months, they would present her with a treatment plan. Joyce chose to continue with her professional/prescription home care program.

8/23/11: Joyce came in today for a hygiene appointment, but it had been almost 12 months since her last appointment. She shared that her employer had laid her off, and while she had not been in for a cleaning and examination, she had continued to come in to the office to pick up her home care products and had not missed a day on the home care program. Her three risk factors of frequent snacking, drinks other than water more than 2 times daily, and daily medications (oral contraceptive and acid reflux medication) were still present. Her CariScreen score was 963, which is below the 1500 threshold. As she was paying out of pocket for this appointment, she was so relieved to hear that her investment in her home care program had paid off and that she had no new cavities and required no additional restorations. She informed her dentist that, at this time, she could not afford the cosmetic restorations she wanted but had a lead on a great job and was planning to be able to look into it in the next year. Her dentist said that he would like to see her continue her low-risk status with no new decay for another 12 months before they could begin that process anyway, and that she just needed to keep up her home care program with the rinse and gel that contained an antibacterial (0.2% sodium hypochlorite), fluoride, xylitol, pH neutralization, and nanoparticles of hydroxyapatite for remineralization support. But she no longer needed to wear the gel in a tray at night. She was committed to the program and so glad she had chosen to come to this dental practice and had saved her teeth and was no longer discussing dentures at all.

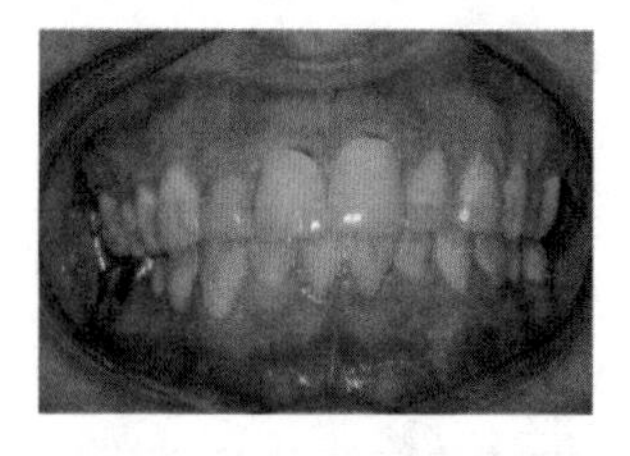

5/15/12: Joyce was in for another cleaning and exam appointment. Her x-rays and examination showed no new decay. It had been 9 months since her last appointment, and she had a new job as an accounts manager for a distribution company, and her responsibilities were primarily to make phone calls to current accounts. While she loved her new job, she really was looking forward to getting back to the face-to-face sales positions she had previously enjoyed. Her three risk factors of frequent snacking, drinks other than water more than 2 times daily, and daily medications (oral contraceptive and acid reflux medication) were still present. Her CariScreen score was 1362, and she had no new decay. Her dentist was very impressed with her adherence to the home care program, and she had been diligent every day since her first appointment for his recommended therapy. Joyce and her dentist decided it was time to set an appointment to discuss her cosmetic restorative options. She was ecstatic that she finally, after a lifetime of battling with dental decay, was going to have the Hollywood smile she had always wanted and would probably never have to have another conversation about dentures with her dentist again. She was continuing with her dentist's recommended caries therapy advice and, since her first appointment, had referred over 65 of her friends, family, and clients to her dentist for caries risk assessment. The dentist knew each and every patient Joyce had referred because she continued to tell everyone she knew: "They saved me!"

Step 7:

Selecting the Proper Treatment Strategy

The primary goal when selecting the proper treatment strategy is to provide enough protective agents to outweigh any risk factors or biofilm challenge present and reverse the balance back toward health. This involves choosing specific treatment agents targeted to offset specific issues. For example, if a patient is screened and a high biofilm challenge (bacterial infection) is identified, a broad-spectrum oxidizing antibacterial agent capable of penetrating a biofilm (0.2% sodium hypochlorite) should be part of the treatment strategy.

Based on each patient's specific level of risk, the patient will be offered three different choices with regard to initial therapy. A "recommended therapy," which is designed to provide enough protective factors to outweigh each patient's specific risk level and move them toward an oral health balance. A "provisional therapy," which is a lower-cost alternative to the recommended therapy and designed to provide enough protective factors to simply keep a patient from getting worse assuming no increase in risk factors. The "provisional therapy" will likely not outweigh the patient's risk. As a third option, the patient can choose to decline any recommended changes. With each option, the patient can be informed of the likelihood that they will experience new decay in the next 12 months if they continue with their current behavioral/diet/home care habits (e.g., high/extreme-risk patients have an 88% chance of experiencing new decay in the next 12 months without a change in care).

The Caries Management Guide (See Figure 17) provides the general guidelines for managing caries risk based on each patient's specific risk assessment. Here are some more specific recommendations based on different types of risk factors or issues a patient may face.

Rev8- 3

CARIES MANAGEMENT GUIDE

1 LOW RISK	2 MODERATE RISK	3 HIGH RISK	4 HIGH RISK	5 HIGH/EXTREME RISK
No Risk Factors No Disease Indicators Low Biofilm Challenge	Risk Factors No Disease Indicators Low Biofilm Challenge	Risk Factors No Disease Indicators High Biofilm Challenge	Risk Factors Disease Indicators Low Biofilm Challenge	Risk Factors Disease Indicators High Biofilm Challenge
RECOMMENDED THERAPY				
Therapy Optional CTx12 Kit *~3 month supply* *$45* 3 CTx4 Gel 5000 Reassess in 6-12 months	CTx12 Kit *~3 month supply* *$45* 3 CTx4 Gel 5000 Modify risk factors Reassess/refill in 3 months	CTx26 Kit *~3 month supply* *$99* 2 CTx4 Treatment Rinse 2 CTx3 Rinse 3 CTx4 Gel 5000 Modify risk factors Reassess/refill in 3 months	CTx21 Kit *~3 month supply* *$69* 3 CTx3 Rinse 3 CTx4 Gel 5000 Modify risk factors Reassess/refill in 3 months	CTx36 Kit *~3 month supply* *$149* 6 CTx4 Treatment Rinse 3 CTx4 Gel 5000 Modify risk factors Reassess/refill in 3 months
PROVISIONAL THERAPY				
Therapy Optional Reassess in 6-12 months	Therapy Optional Reassess in 6 months	CTx21 Kit *~3 month supply* *$69* 3 CTx3 Rinse 3 CTx4 Gel 5000 Modify risk factors Reassess/refill in 6 months	CTx12 Kit *~3 month supply* *$45* 3 CTx4 Gel 5000 Modify risk factors Reassess/refill in 3 months	CTx26 Kit *~3 month supply* *$99* 2 CTx4 Treatment Rinse 2 CTx3 Rinse 3 CTx4 Gel 5000 Modify risk factors Reassess/refill in 3 months
DECLINE				
23.6% risk of new cavities within 1 year[1]	38.6% risk of new cavities within 1 year[1]	38.6 - 69.3% risk of new cavities within 1 year[1]	69.3% risk of new cavities within 1 year[1]	88% risk of new cavities within 1 year[1]

With all therapy options, significant time and effort are required; however, the benefits are worthwhile when you choose to take steps toward improving your health.

[1]Validation of the CDA CAMBRA Caries Risk Assessment - A Six-Year Retrospective Study; Doméjean, White and Featherstone; CDA Journal, October 2011

It is also recommended to follow the ADA Council of Scientific Affairs Recommendations for Pit and Fissure Sealants, the ADA Council of Scientific Affairs Topical Fluoride Recommendations based on Caries Risk, and the FDA Guidelines for Prescribing Dental Radiographs based on Caries Risk

Figure 17. Example of a Caries Management Guide, courtesy of carifree.com

Risk Factors

"I notice plaque buildup on my teeth between brushings." Rapid growth of the bacterial biofilm between brushings may be a sign of inadequate home care, inadequate oral care product selection, low saliva flow, or frequent consumption of food and drink providing additional nutrients to the biofilm, stimulating growth. Elevated pH (8.0+) dental products (gels, sprays, rinses) should be considered to offset the potential acidic side effects of the excessive plaque biofilm. Broad-spectrum oxidizing antibacterial rinses (0.2% sodium hypochlorite) should also be considered to lower the total bacterial load.

"Do you take medications daily? If so, how many?" Taking just one medication daily can affect saliva flow, and most people may not even notice. Taking multiple medications can compound the salivary flow issue. Elevated pH (8.0+) dental products with xylitol in the form of gels or sprays should be considered after meals and snacks to quickly elevate the pH after an acid challenge. Depending on the patient's caries risk, prescription/professional home care products for brushing and rinsing should be considered.

"Do you feel you have a dry mouth at any time of the day or night?" If you are noticing a dry mouth at any time, the problem of saliva flow should be a serious concern. By the time the patient notices a saliva flow problem, the problem is likely severe. Elevated pH (8.0+) dental products with xylitol in the form of gels or sprays are essential after meals and snacks to quickly elevate the pH after an acid challenge. Elevated pH gels with xylitol and nanohydroxyapatite can be worn in whitening trays at night if nighttime oral dryness is an issue. Depending on the patient's caries risk, prescription/professional products with pH neutralization, xylitol, fluoride, and nanohydroxyapatite for morning and night home care should be prescribed.

"Do you drink liquids other than water more than 2 times daily between meals?" Every time a patient drinks something other than water between meals, they are adding an additional daily acid attack on their teeth. This acid attack can increase cavity-causing bacterial growth as well as supply the current biofilm with additional nutrients, creating acids that demineralize the teeth. If the patient is not willing to change this dietary habit or move their beverage consumption to meal times, elevated pH (8.0+) dental products with xylitol in the form of gels or sprays should be considered after meals and drinks to quickly elevate the pH after an acid challenge. Depending on the patient's caries risk, prescription/professional home care products for brushing and rinsing should be considered.

"Do you snack daily between meals?" Every time a patient eats something (yes, even nuts, fruits, and vegetables), they are adding an additional daily acid attack on their teeth. This acid attack can increase cavity-causing bacterial growth as well as supply the current biofilm with additional nutrients, creating acids that demineralize the teeth. If the patient is not willing to change this dietary habit or it is something necessary for their health, elevated pH (8.0+) dental products with xylitol in the form of gels or sprays should be considered after snacks to quickly elevate the pH after an acid challenge. Depending on the patient's caries risk, prescription/professional home care products for brushing and rinsing should be considered.

"Do you have an oral appliance present?" Oral appliances create artificial areas on the teeth that can not only be hard to clean but also allow a biofilm to mature and potentially demineralize teeth. Patients with oral appliances should be aware of other risk factors and consider using a broad-spectrum oxidizing antibacterial agent capable of penetrating a biofilm to help reduce biofilm in areas that are hard to reach with brushing and flossing. Elevated pH (8.0+) dental care products with 1.1% neutral sodium fluoride, xylitol, and nanoparticles of hydroxyapatite should also be considered to support remineralization.

"Other health concerns." Other health concerns such as tobacco use, acid reflux, and diabetes are important as, often, patients with these concerns experience increased acid attacks and/or reduced salivary flow. Elevated pH (8.0+) dental products with xylitol in the form of gels or sprays are essential to quickly elevate the pH after an acid challenge. Elevated pH gels with xylitol and nanohydroxyapatite can be worn in whitening trays at night if oral dryness or excessive acid attacks are an issue. Depending on the patient's caries risk, prescription/professional products with pH neutralization, xylitol, fluoride, and nanohydroxyapatite for morning and night home care should be prescribed.

Disease Indicators

Disease indicators such as new or progressing cavitations, new or progressing white spot lesions, etc., are signs/symptoms of the disease. Patients with signs or symptoms are advised to make changes to their home care product regimen and consider behavioral changes to modify risk factors whenever possible. Put simply, if the patient's current home care product regimen was working and keeping the patient in healthy balance, it would have worked and no changes would be necessary.

Biofilm Challenge

Patients with a high biofilm challenge identified by ATP (CariScreen) testing or by bacterial culture are at increased risk for decay. For this reason, a broad-spectrum oxidizing antibacterial agent capable of penetrating a biofilm, such as 0.2% sodium hypochlorite oral rinse, should be considered as part of a treatment strategy.

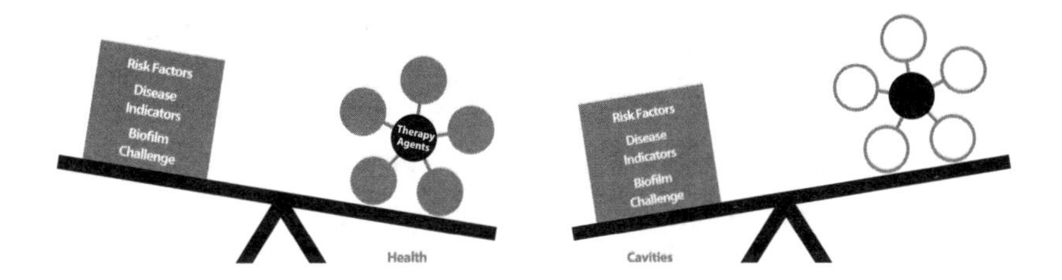

Two opposing caries balances, one where protective factors outweigh risk factors, and one where risk factors outweigh protective factors

Step 8:

Restorative Care

Dental caries is a disease that leads to net mineral loss of the teeth and, in many instances, cavitation and lesions of the teeth. Early mineral loss will display as white spot lesions, and more advanced mineral loss will present as cavitated lesions. The research is clear that noncavitated or white spot lesions need not and should not be restored. What used to be considered the "ideal board exam lesion," an E2 lesion, is not cavitated 85% of the time, and the first approach to therapy should be remineralization of the lesion.[69] Smooth surface white spot lesions need to be categorized into active and inactive or remineralized lesions. The surface of an active smooth surface white spot lesion is dull or chalky in appearance when air from a three-way syringe is blown across it. The inactive or remineralized smooth surface white spot lesion remains shiny in surface appearance when air is similarly blown over it. All active noncavitated white spot lesions should be remineralized with professional/prescription therapy, including fluoride. Cavitated smooth surface lesions need to be restored. This leads to the question, when in the overall therapeutic process should cavitated lesions be restored, and what materials should be used?

The research is not clear on whether it is best to restore the cavitated lesions first and then treat the patient with antimicrobial/anticaries therapy if indicated, or if it is best to treat the patient with anticaries therapies first and then restore the cavitated lesions. Ultimately, to reduce the cariogenic pathogens successfully, the lesions act as a source of this infection and need to be eliminated. It makes sense to both accomplish the anticaries therapy and restore any cavitated lesions simultaneously, recognizing that it may take staging multiple restorative appointments over the span of a month, while the anticaries therapy may be ongoing for 3–6 months or more.

The restorative material of choice becomes the next issue. For high/extreme-risk patients, placing expensive final restorative materials such as crowns, veneers, or final composites at the time of initially removing the cavitated lesions comes with the risk that these restorations may fail, depending on the patient's adherence to the anticaries therapy. Additionally, depending on the size and the extent of the lesions, combined with the patient's overall risk status and severity of risk factors and disease indicators, the clinician and patient might be better off by restoring the lesions initially with GIC (glass ionomer cement) materials until the patient is at lower caries risk for a period of a year or more. The GIC material provides the added benefit of acting as a fluoride reservoir in the mouth and will transport fluoride ions into the enamel and dentin. Then once the patient has been low/moderate risk and decay free for a period of a year or longer, definitive final restorations can be placed with reduced risk of failure due to secondary decay. If the patient has dental insurance, this creates an additional dilemma. While the teeth will essentially be restored twice in the span of a couple of years, the insurance plan may only provide a benefit for restoring them once. In most situations like this, it is common practice for the practitioner to give the patient the option of utilizing their insurance benefit for the provisional (short-term) restorations or the final restorations and recognize that the patient will be paying for one set of restorations.

A patient may opt to have the final restorations placed at the initial decay removal stage, but needs to be fully informed of the risk of recurring decay around these newly placed restorations during the process of creating a healthy balance in their mouth. If the patient chooses this option, *they need to be willing to assume the responsibility of any restoration failure*, recognizing that restoration failure due to recurring decay is not the fault or responsibility of the dental practitioner.

If the patient chooses this option, they need to be willing to assume the responsibility of any restoration failure...

Step 9:

Treatment Expectations (How long does treatment take?)

There are many confounding factors that influence caries risk treatment time and the potential results a patient and practitioner can expect. Each patient's oral biofilm is as uniquely specific to them as -their fingerprint, and no two patients will respond exactly alike to therapy and remineralization agents. It is important to remember that high-risk patients may require therapy modification throughout the treatment phase to reach a state of balance. Many patients may require ongoing therapy agent usage during the maintenance phase. Perhaps for life, if risk factors are unmodifiable or still present. The good news is that professional/prescription dental products have also improved at treating both the pH imbalance and the bacterial condition that may be present. Professional/prescription products are also capable of remineralization under the right conditions. Take-home professional therapy should be recommended in 3- to 6-month increments, and reassessment should take place as soon as the prescribed therapy is finished.

Factors Influencing Treatment Time and Results

Time. The length of time a patient has been experiencing issues with dental decay should be considered when setting therapy expectations. A patient who has experienced symptoms of the imbalance (cavities) for years is probably going to require more therapy over a longer period of time than a patient with their first cavity. This is why caries risk assessment is vital. The earlier a patient can be identified at risk, and the sooner intervention can be initiated, the shorter the duration of treatment will likely be.

Number of risk factors. The number of risk factors plays an important role in treatment time and effort. Patients with multiple risk factors will likely face a greater challenge to lower their risk and reduce the incidence of signs/symptoms than patients with one risk factor. Many risk factors, when combined, can cause a compounding effect on a patient's risk. For example, frequent snacking combined with low saliva flow can make the acid challenges a patient experiences longer and more intense, placing a greater challenge on the effectiveness of therapeutic agents and strategies. The more risk factors a patient has, the more therapy may be required.

Modifiable versus unmodifiable risk factors. If the risk factors driving the disease progression for a patient are unmodifiable, such as life-requiring prescription medications that cause reduced salivary flow, it will increase the length of time a patient will require therapy. If the risk factors driving the patient's disease are behavioral habits, and the patient is not yet ready to change those behaviors, more therapy and time may be required. Modifying and eliminating risk factors is the most cost-effective method of therapy, and an essential part of reducing a patient's caries risk.

Risk factor severity. Patients may need to rely on their dental professionals' expertise to define the severity of specific risk factors, such as salivary flow or biofilm challenge. As an example, a patient taking a single medication daily (while it is an important risk factor to consider) is probably not as severe as a patient taking ten different types of medications daily. For some patients, the severity of their risk factors can create a dramatic barrier to reaching a state of oral health balance.

Risk factor frequency. The frequency a patient is being exposed to risk factors should be analyzed when considering treatment time and expectations. If a patient is consuming one snack per day, the frequency may not be of as much concern as a patient who snacks 3 or more times per day between meals. Patients who are experiencing a higher frequency of exposure to risk factors will require more time and effort to reach a state of oral health balance.

Presence of symptoms. If a patient's disease has progressed to the point of experiencing signs/symptoms of the oral imbalance such as visible cavitations, white spot lesions, or cavities identified on x-rays, they have reached a later stage of the disease and have a longer treatment time than a patient who has yet to express signs/symptoms.

Severity of signs/symptoms. The severity of the signs/symptoms should also be an indicator of the amount of time and effort required to reach a state of oral health balance. A patient with one new cavity is not in as severe a condition as a patient with several new cavities.

Timely restorations. The capability of therapy products to modify a biofilm and help move a patient toward health will be hindered by unrestored sites of disease. While remineralization is possible for early lesions that have not progressed beyond the DEJ (dentin-enamel junction), or E2 lesions, once the lesion depth has penetrated the DEJ and is a D1 or D2 lesion, the enamel surface is cavitated and the tooth requires surgical removal of the lesion followed by restoration. Cavitations that have reached a depth requiring restoration must be restored in a timely manner, and potential sources of the infection must be removed, if an oral health balance is to be achieved.

Level of therapy. Patients have choices when moving forward with prescription/professional therapy, and the level of therapy they choose partially dictates the length and expectations of therapy. For example, if the recommended therapy for a high/extreme-risk patient is a professional home care kit for 3 months, and the patient chooses an over-the-counter preparation, the patient's expectations need to be appropriately adjusted. The patient may experience no change or only experience a slowing progression of signs/symptoms or biofilm challenge rather than a meaningful reduction or reversal. However, choosing to do something rather than doing nothing is always a smarter move toward health.

Patient therapy compliance/adherence/participation. While it may seem fundamental, lack of patient follow-through with medical recommendations is one of the primary reasons diagnosed medical conditions continue to progress. The majority of prescriptions written in the United States never even make it to the pharmacy to get filled, much less get taken on a regular basis as prescribed. It is essential that patients continue to use the therapy they have been prescribed, as prescribed, for the duration of the therapy time recommended. If the patient has been prescribed 3 months of therapy product but reassessment with their dentist has not been scheduled for 6 months, the patient should get another 3-month supply as directed after the initial therapy product has been used, or risk regression of their disease risk status.

Therapy Milestones and What to Do

Assuming a patient has chosen to move forward with some form of therapy or preventive product with pH neutralization, 0.2% sodium hypochlorite, 0.5% or 1.1% fluoride, xylitol, and nanoparticles of hydroxyapatite and the therapy has been supplied in 3-month increments, it is advisable to reperform a full caries risk assessment and each subsequent reassessment appointment at 3-month intervals. The number, frequency, and severity of risk factors can change substantially between appointments.

Three months. Depending on the level and severity of the patient's risk, some practitioners may wish to reassess the patients risk and therapy level at 3 months, while most have the patient continue the therapy for 6 months. Many patients (if compliant) show some form of progress at the 3-month appointment (See Figure 18). Although it may not be enough to lower the patient's therapy requirements yet, the progress can encourage both the patient and the practitioner that the patient is on the right therapy program. Some examples of progress might be remineralization of early white spot lesions or areas of demineralization, improved visual soft tissue health and appearance, decrease in bleeding gums when flossing or probing, reduction in sensitivity, decreased incidence of halitosis (bad breath), a feeling of "cleaner" teeth, reduced noticeable plaque buildup, "hardening" of tooth enamel, improved tooth luster, etc. Some patients with a high biofilm challenge at the initial appointment may see a reduction in their biofilm challenge at the 3-month reassessment. The patients likely to see a reduction in their biofilm challenge at this point are patients that initially presented with limited risk factors, no severe risk factors, and no disease indicators and who were compliant with professional recommendations.

Reduced biofilm challenge/plaque build-up
Lower CariScreen ATP test or CFU's by culture
Lower decay rate
Remineralization of early white spot lesions or areas of demineralization
Improved visual soft tissue health and appearance
Decrease in bleeding gums when flossing or probing
Reduction in sensitivity
Decreased incidence of halitosis (bad breath)
A feeling of "cleaner" teeth
Reduced noticeable plaque buildup
"Hardening" of tooth enamel
Improved tooth luster

Figure 18. Examples of caries therapy progress

A practitioner's goal at the 3-month reassessment should be to identify any kind of progress and verify patient participation or compliance. If progress is identified, it is recommended that the patient continue with the current level of therapy. If no progress is identified, it is recommended that the patient either increase their level of therapy, continue with the current level of therapy with modified expectations, or continue with the current level of therapy and modify one risk factor.

Six months. Most patients (if compliant) will show progress at the 6-month appointment, and the progress may be adequate to lower the patient's therapy level. Some examples of progress might be remineralization of early areas of demineralization, improved soft tissue health on inspection, decrease in bleeding gums when flossing or probing, reduction in sensitivity, decreased incidence of halitosis (bad breath), feeling of "cleaner" teeth, reduced plaque buildup, "hardening" of tooth enamel, improved tooth luster, and/or reduced incidence of cavities. Some patients with a high biofilm challenge at the initial appointment may see a reduction in their biofilm challenge at the 6-month reassessment. The patients most likely to see a reduction in their biofilm challenge at this point are patients that initially presented with limited risk factors, no severe risk factors, and no disease indicators or limited disease indicators.

A practitioner's goal at the 6-month reassessment should be to identify progress of any kind, verify adherence, and if the practitioner or patient is not satisfied with the progress, recommend an increase in the patient's level of therapy. If the patient assesses at a lower level of risk, suggest the recommended level of therapy for that new risk level and caution the patient that relapse is a possible outcome until multiple healthy appointments have been established. Therapy recommendations should be made for the next 6 months. Keep in mind during these reassessment appointments the factors influencing treatment time and results such as the amount of time the patient has had the issue; the number, frequency, and severity of risk factors; the presence and severity of symptoms; the restorative treatment plan; and the level of compliance.

Twelve months. Approximately 80–90% of compliant patients will see substantial progress by the 12-month appointment. Examples of progress would be reduced progression of biofilm challenge or decay, lower incidence of decay, lower biofilm challenge (See Figure 19), improved soft tissue health on inspection, decrease in bleeding gums when flossing or probing, improved enamel luster, reduced plaque buildup, etc. Patients who may have yet to see substantial progress are patients with severe or unmodifiable risk factors, patients who were not successfully adherent or have gaps in their treatment regimen, and patients with a long history of severe decay.

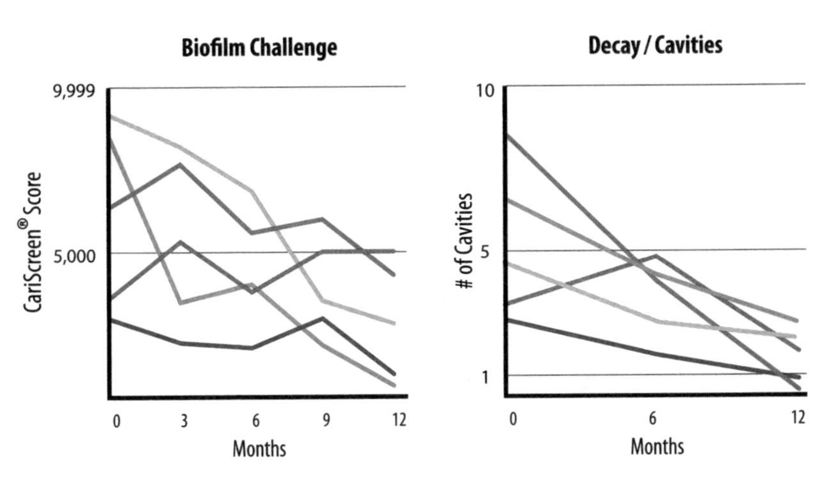

Figure 19. Examples of reduced progression of biofilm challenge and decay after 12 months of therapy

Again, the practitioner's goal at the 12-month reassessment should be to identify progress of any kind and verify adherence to the recommended therapeutic regimen. If the practitioner or patient is not satisfied with the progress, there should be a recommendation to increase the patient's level of therapy. If the patient has been assessed at a lower level of risk, suggest the recommended level of therapy for that new risk level and caution the patient that relapse is a possible outcome until multiple healthy appointments have been established. Therapy recommendations should be made for the next 6 months. Keep in mind during these reassessment appointments the factors influencing treatment time and results such as the amount of time the patient has had the issue; the number, frequency, and severity of risk factors; the presence and severity of symptoms; the restorative treatment plan; and the level of participation or adherence.

Reassessment Tip

It is important to note that the 3-, 6-, and 12-month appointments are very critical tipping points for patients looking to improve their level of health and reduce their risk. The practitioner must work with the patient to determine realistic expectations based on the choices the patient makes and how that corresponds with the patient's disease condition and long-term goals. Historically, many patients and practitioners have the impression that treatment of medical conditions is one of quick fixes with a simple pill, and the expectation of immediate results. But the oral imbalance/infection that causes dental decay is one that often begins in the patient's first months of life and may take long periods of time to manifest and consequently can take significant time and effort to reverse. Many patients and practitioners have expectations that prescription/professional oral care products can work similarly to antibiotics given to a patient with a minor infection such as an ear infection, and if the patient is compliant with the prescription, the problem will clear up in 10–14 days. This is not the case with dental caries, a complex, multifactorial biofilm and pH specific disease.

The reality of therapy expectations for dental disease should be closer in comparison to weight loss. While it can take only a few months to put on an unhealthy amount of weight, the work and time required to lose the weight may be longer and require more time and effort. Similarly, the longer a patient has had a weight problem, the longer it may take them to reach their goals and relapse is common. Many patients and practitioners choose to wait until there are serious signs/symptoms of the problem, such as cavities, prior to making changes to behavioral risk factors or prescribing targeted oral care therapy products. The sooner patients can be identified with risk factors or a biofilm challenge prior to cavities developing, the less time and effort it will take to get the patient back into balance.

For patients looking to begin a weight loss program, there are generally three ways they can choose to move forward. They can begin an exercise program while making no dietary changes. They can make dietary changes while making no changes to their activity level. Or they can increase their level of exercise *and* make dietary changes. Each and every patient is different, and how they choose to attack the issue will be based on their individual issues and goals. But patients that make consistent changes over time on both sides of the equation will experience the most success.

Patients with high caries risk have the same variety of options when the goal is achieving a healthy oral balance. On one side of the equation, they can choose to make behavioral changes and reduce their risk factors while continuing their current oral care product and hygiene regimen. Another option is to make no changes to their behavioral risk factors and make changes to their hygiene regimen with prescription/professional oral care products. Ideally, patients at risk would choose to alter their oral care product and hygiene regimen *as well as* the modifiable behavioral risk factors associated with the disease. But behavioral studies have shown that the most successful patients choose to make one lifestyle change at a time; and it is recommended that at each stage of the 3-, 6-, and 12-month appointments, patients and practitioners choose only one area at a time to modify. During the process, based on each reassessment, they can additionally decide if more changes are necessary based on the progress made. When there are several different behaviors that should be changed, it is advisable to offer the options to the patient and let them pick the behavior they want to focus on.

Finally, patients and practitioners must be looking not only for obvious signs of progress but also for a reduction in the progression of the disease.

Just as a patient who is beginning a weight loss program and has a history of gaining additional weight every month and with diet modification may at first see only a slowing of the additional weight gain, a dental patient who has had a history of high biofilm challenge may only experience a slight decrease in the elevation path of the biofilm challenge at first, or only experience a reduction in the number of new cavities they develop. Instead of developing 2 or 3 new cavities every year, they may only develop 1 new cavity. Although these patients are continuing to see progression of the disease, they are making progress and should be encouraged to continue making changes to reach their goals.

Eighteen to thirty-six months. 90+% of compliant patients see substantial progress if they continue with therapy for 36 months. Examples of progress would be reduced progression of biofilm challenge, lower decay rate or eliminated incidence of decay, lower biofilm challenge, improved soft tissue health on inspection, decrease in bleeding gums when flossing or probing, improved enamel luster, reduced plaque buildup, etc.

Again, the practitioner's goal at the 18- to 36-month reassessments should be to identify progress of any kind, verify compliance, and if the practitioner or patient is not satisfied with the progress, increase the patient's level of therapy. If the patient assessed is at a lower level of risk, suggest the recommended level of therapy for that new risk level and caution the patient that relapse is a possible outcome until multiple healthy appointments have been established. Therapy recommendations should be made for the next 6 months. Keep in mind during these reassessment appointments the factors influencing treatment time and results such as the amount of time the patient has had the issue; the number, frequency, and severity of risk factors; the presence and severity of symptoms; the restorative treatment plan; and the level of compliance.

Patients who, by the 36-month appointment, are still experiencing dental decay are those that were noncompliant with therapy, noncompliant with behavioral risk factor changes, patients who have gaps in their treatment regimen, or patients with a long history of severe decay or have severe and unmodifiable risk factors. Many of these patients can and will reach a level of balance with their oral health, but for some, that level of balance may be one with a reduced but still occurring level of decay or a plateaued but elevated biofilm challenge.

Step 10:

Long-Term Maintenance

One of most common questions regarding caries management therapy is, "Will the patient need to be on therapy products for life?" Like most medical questions, the answer is never black-and-white and every patient is different. For this reason, in conjunction with members of the Western, Central, and Eastern CAMBRA Coalitions, a Caries Management Guide (See Figure 20) was developed to provide direction for both the practitioner and the patient on what level of therapy is necessary at each level of risk as patients move their personal balance toward health.

Rev8-3

CARIES MANAGEMENT GUIDE

No Risk Factors No Disease Indicators Low Biofilm Challenge 1 LOW RISK	Risk Factors No Disease Indicators Low Biofilm Challenge 2 MODERATE RISK	Risk Factors No Disease Indicators High Biofilm Challenge 3 HIGH RISK	Risk Factors Disease Indicators Low Biofilm Challenge 4 HIGH RISK	Risk Factors Disease Indicators High Biofilm Challenge 5 HIGH/EXTREME RISK
RECOMMENDED THERAPY				
Therapy Optional CTx12 Kit ~3 month supply $45 3 CTx4 Gel 5000 Reassess in 6-12 months	CTx12 Kit ~3 month supply $45 3 CTx4 Gel 5000 Modify risk factors Reassess/refill in 3 months	CTx26 Kit ~3 month supply $99 2 CTx4 Treatment Rinse 2 CTx3 Rinse 3 CTx4 Gel 5000 Modify risk factors Reassess/refill in 3 months	CTx21 Kit ~3 month supply $69 3 CTx3 Rinse 3 CTx4 Gel 5000 Modify risk factors Reassess/refill in 3 months	CTx36 Kit ~3 month supply $149 6 CTx4 Treatment Rinse 3 CTx4 Gel 5000 Modify risk factors Reassess/refill in 3 months
PROVISIONAL THERAPY				
Therapy Optional Reassess in 6-12 months	Therapy Optional Reassess in 6 months	CTx21 Kit ~3 month supply $69 3 CTx3 Rinse 3 CTx4 Gel 5000 Modify risk factors Reassess/refill in 6 months	CTx12 Kit ~3 month supply $45 3 CTx4 Gel 5000 Modify risk factors Reassess/refill in 3 months	CTx26 Kit ~3 month supply $99 2 CTx4 Treatment Rinse 2 CTx3 Rinse 3 CTx4 Gel 5000 Modify risk factors Reassess/refill in 3 months
DECLINE				
23.6% risk of new cavities within 1 year[1]	38.6% risk of new cavities within 1 year[1]	38.6 - 69.3% risk of new cavities within 1 year[1]	69.3% risk of new cavities within 1 year[1]	88% risk of new cavities within 1 year[1]
With all therapy options, significant time and effort are required; however, the benefits are worthwhile when you choose to take steps toward improving your health.				

[1]Validation of the CDA CAMBRA Caries Risk Assessment - A Six-Year Retrospective Study; Doméjean, White and Featherstone; CDA Journal, October 2011
It is also recommended to follow the ADA Council of Scientific Affairs Recommendations for Pit and Fissure Sealants, the ADA Council of Scientific Affairs Topical Fluoride Recommendations based on Caries Risk, and the FDA Guidelines for Prescribing Dental Radiographs based on Caries Risk

Figure 20. Example of a Caries Management Guide, courtesy of carifree.com

The short answer to the long-term maintenance question is to follow the Caries Management Guide and, based on each patient's specific risk assessment, follow the recommendations provided. For some patients who, with therapy, eliminate many of the factors driving their disease, they will move to a lower risk category. Low and moderate caries risk patients have choices within the Caries Management Guide to opt out of using any professional / prescription therapy products and use common over-the-counter dental products designed for low-risk patients. Moderate- and high-caries-risk patients with unmodifiable risk factors may have ongoing need for continued professional / prescription therapy products and strategies.

The Science of ATP Testing (CariScreen)

ATP stands for adenosine triphosphate and is the energy molecule in all living cells. In the mouth, ATP provides the opportunity to measure bacterial load and biofilm activity levels as they relate to health. ATP bioluminescence testing is the method for rapidly measuring the quantity of microorganisms through the detection of adenosine triphosphate. ATP is quantified by measuring the light produced through its reaction with the naturally occurring firefly enzyme "luciferase" using a luminometer, a very sensitive light measuring device. ATP testing has been used in a variety of health and biologic testing methods since the 1960s but has only in the last 10 years been adapted to dentistry and dental caries diagnosis.

$$ATP + O_2 + luciferin \xrightarrow{Mg^{++}\ luciferase} AMP + PPi - oxyluciferin + light$$

One of the primary issues related to dental microbiological testing has been the sheer number of bacterial species implicated in the disease process. Until recently, dental caries was thought to be a fairly simple disease. It was thought to be caused primarily by two bacteria, *Mutans streptococci* and *Lactobacillus*[70, 71] and required only refined sugar and tooth structure to occur. The traditional disease model was supported by an abundance of scientific studies linking *Mutans streptococci* and *Lactobacillus* levels to caries risk in children.[72, 73] But as the field of biofilm research developed, a broader, more complex picture became apparent. More bacteria were implicated in the disease process by different researchers worldwide.[74] Now oral biofilms can be studied with forensic-type precision by identifying the bacteria with the 16S gene sequence of their rRNA.[75] This has added additional species to the growing list of bacterial species now implicated in the dental decay process (See Figure 21).[76, 77, 78, 79, 80, 81, 82, 83, 84, 85, 86, 87, 88]

BACTERIA IMPLICATED IN DENTAL CARIES

BACTERIAL SPP.	AUTHORS										
	Beighton	Hayes	van Houte	Becker	Loesche	Hamada	Kleinberg	Bunting	Tanner	Hoshino	Sissons
Streptococcus salivarius	●			●							
S. parasanguinis				●							●
S. constellatus				●							
S. mutans		●	●	●	●	●	●				●
S. sobrinus			●		●	●	●				
S. oralis	●		●				●				●
S. milleri			●								
S. mitis			●								●
S. gordonii			●								
S. anginosus			●								
S. cricetus							●				
S. intermedius									●		●
Lactobacillus fermentum				●							●
L. plantarum										●	●
L. acidophilus							●	●			
L. casei							●				
Candida albicans						●					●
Actinomyces israelii	●										●
A. gerensceriae	●			●							
A. naeslundii	●										
Veillonella				●							
Veillonella parvula							●				
Bifidobacterium			●	●							
Neisseria sicca							●				
Fusobacterium animalis				●							
Capnocytophaga gingivalis											●
S. vestibularis											●

***These bacterial species are related to caries as per the author's interpretation after reading articles by the listed authors.*

Figure 21. Bacterial species implicated in the caries disease process

A Clinical Look at CAMBRA, Dental Products Report August 2007. Kutsch, V., Kutsch, C., and Nelson, B. C.

Recent biofilm research based on 16S gene sequence DNA evidence is also broadening the picture of dental caries. It is clear now that some of the previous paradigms on the microbiology of dental caries were wrong.[84, 89] The mouth represents a unique environment in the body for biofilms. The teeth are the only nonshedding surfaces in the body, so the biofilms on the teeth tend to be more complex and microbiologically diverse than previously thought.[90] While more than 700 bacterial phylotypes could potentially be found in the human mouth, a healthy individual only has around 113 different bacterial species, while a high-caries-risk individual has an average of 94, presumably because fewer bacteria are capable of surviving the low pH conditions consistent with the disease.[91]

Based on the biofilm disease model, with a large number of different species of bacteria participating in the disease process and high (100 times) usage of ATP being one of the common "fingerprints" of aciduric bacteria, a better metric of assessment is ATP testing.[92] The survival of acidogenic/aciduric (cavity-causing) bacteria depends on their ability to produce enough ATP to effectively transport the H+ (acidic) ions out of the cell, thereby maintaining intracellular neutrality necessary for survival.[93] The concept of ATP bioluminescence has been tested with strong positive correlation values in dental caries risk assessment and fits the nonspecific bacterial biofilm model.[92]

Even with all of this evidence, one common misconception is that all patients with current decay will test high with ATP bioluminescence testing. The reality is high levels of bacteria are not always the primary factor driving dental decay. Dental caries is a multifactorial pH dysfunction disease. For some patients, a highly destructive diet may be the primary driver. For others, it may be poor-quality saliva or poor saliva flow making them more susceptible. The purpose of ATP testing is *not* to identify "bacterial challenge" or "biofilm challenge" as the sole factor responsible for a patient's disease, but rather either include it as one of the multiple factors associated with a patient's condition when making treatment, restorative, and cosmetic recommendations, or eliminate it, allowing patients and practitioners to focus on other factors involved.

Dental Insurance and Caries Management by Risk Assessment (CAMBRA)

There are many misconceptions within the public perception of dentistry surrounding dental insurance. The first and most important is the idea that "dental insurance" is "insurance" at all. When individuals purchase "insurance," the purpose is primarily to protect themselves from an unlikely event or situation that would cost a significant amount of money—for example, the loss of a house in a fire, or being diagnosed with cancer requiring hundreds of thousands of dollars in medical procedures. This is true for most types of insurance as the insurance company collects small monthly premiums from a large number of participants and pays out loss-connected benefits according to their policies on statistically rare events or situations. This is the true definition of insurance. Fire insurance, life insurance, homeowner's insurance, and even medical insurance all come under this definition.

A better definition of dental insurance is that it is more of a "dental benefit." Dentistry is not a rare event, and according to the CDC, 85% of all adults experience dental decay. The cost of this care, while it is not inexpensive, does not accumulate to the levels of unexpected surgery and a long-term medical stay or replacing a home. Consequently, the classic model of insurance doesn't work well in dentistry. For that reason, in the 1960s, dental insurance was invented as an employer-sponsored benefit to assist employees in offsetting the costs of regular dental maintenance. But because so many individuals have dental needs, in order to offer the dental insurance, caps were put in place to limit the benefit to $1,000–$2,000 per year in most cases.

Due to this cap, most policies that are purchased by individuals, employers, and employees primarily include coverage for regular cleaning visits and restorative work like fillings and crowns. Although policies do exist with coverage for preventive therapies and other necessary dental procedures, often, dental customers choose insurance policies with a focus on restorative and regular checkup benefits based on a treatment model of care, not a wellness model.

The next most prominent misconception regarding dental insurance occurs when patients believe that their dental benefit covers *all* of their necessary oral health care needs, and anything that is not covered by their benefit is not necessary to maintain their oral health. This is often a real frustration for both dental practitioners and patients. For example, a patient presents with 4 new cavities and periodontal (gum) disease and has caries risk factors and a high biofilm challenge (caries infection). In order to adequately treat the patient and make strides toward health, all areas of decay need to be removed and filled, periodontal therapy performed, and antibacterial caries therapy started. But the patient only has enough dental benefits to cover 2 of the 4 necessary fillings and does not want to move forward with any treatment that is not covered by their benefit.

While "out of pocket" financial implications of dental and medical treatment are always a consideration, and for some, the costs are an insurmountable obstacle, untreated dental disease and untreated oral infections like periodontal disease and caries are *extremely* unlikely to "heal" on their own. Patients who do not take immediate action to repair and treat the disease, or allow their dental benefits to guide their treatment plan, will face amplified progression of the disease and increased costs. For some patients, this is a frustrating downward spiral, and eventually, they reach a "point of no return" and opt to have their teeth removed. This entire book is designed to help stop that process.

The truth is that dental insurance is a product, and what type of procedures covered and the limitations of coverage are bundled into different "policies" or packages, which are then sold to employers or individuals. The dental insurance policies are designed to do three important things: The insurance plan must fit the insurance company's financial needs for profitability. The plan must meet the annual policy price points expected by employers, employees, and individuals. And finally, the plan must provide adequate procedure compensation for the provider (dental practice).

Currently, multiple insurance companies sell policies with coverage for dental procedure codes associated with CAMBRA, including "D0425" for caries susceptibility testing (CariScreen), "D1206" for therapeutic applications of fluoride varnish for moderate- or high-caries-risk patients, "D1310" for nutritional counseling for the control of dental disease, and "D9630" for other drugs, medicaments, or fluoride dispensed by the office for at-home use (see chart of all codes). While this list is not all-inclusive and many other CAMBRA procedure codes exist, many patients believe that if their insurance policy doesn't cover caries susceptibility testing or drugs and medicaments dispensed by the practice for the control of dental disease, the recommendations being made are not necessary for health. This is simply not true.

Insurance Billing Codes Related to CAMBRA

D0145. Oral evaluation for a patient under 3 years of age and counseling with primary caregiver.

Diagnostic and preventive services performed for a child under the age of 3, preferably within the first six months of the eruption of the first primary tooth, including recording the oral and physical health history, evaluation of caries susceptibility, development of an appropriate preventive oral health regimen, and communication with and counseling of the child's parent, legal guardian, and / or primary caregiver.

D0415. Collection of microorganisms for culture and sensitivity.

D0417. Collection and preparation of saliva sample for laboratory diagnostic testing.

D0418. Analysis of saliva sample, chemical or biological analysis of saliva sample for diagnostic purposes.

D0421. Genetic test for susceptibility to oral diseases.

Sample collection for the purpose of certified laboratory analysis to detect specific genetic variations associated with increased susceptibility for oral disease such as severe periodontal disease.

D0425. Caries susceptibility tests, diagnostic test for determining a patient's propensity for caries.

D1110. Prophylaxis—adult.

Removal of plaque, calculus, and stains from the tooth structures in the permanent and transitional dentition. It is intended to control local irritational factors.

D1120. Prophylaxis—child.

Removal of plaque, calculus, and stains from the tooth structures in the primary and transitional dentition. It is intended to control local irritational factors.

> *D1206.* Topical application of fluoride varnish. Prescription strength fluoride product designed solely for use in the dental office, delivered to the dentition under the direct supervision of a dental professional. Fluoride must be applied separately from prophylaxis paste.

D1208. Topical application of fluoride.

D1310. Nutritional counseling for control of dental disease.

Counseling on food selection and dietary habits as a part of treatment and control of periodontal disease and caries.

D1320. Tobacco counseling for the control and prevention of oral disease.

Tobacco prevention and cessation services reduce patient risks of developing tobacco-related oral diseases and conditions and improve prognosis for certain dental therapies.

D1330. Oral hygiene instruction.

This may include instructions for home care. Examples include tooth brushing technique, flossing, and use of special oral hygiene aids.

D1351. Sealant—per tooth.

Mechanically and / or chemically prepared enamel surface sealed to prevent decay.

> *D1352.* Preventive resin restoration in a moderate- to high-caries-risk patient's permanent tooth. Conservative restoration of an active cavitated lesion in a pit or fissure that does not extend into dentin; includes placement of a sealant in any radiating noncarious fissures or pits.

D9630. Other drugs and/or medicaments, by report.

Includes, but is not limited to, oral antibiotics, oral analgesics, and topical fluoride dispensed in the office for home use; does not include writing prescriptions.

D9920. Behavior management, by report.

May be reported in addition to treatment provided. Should be reported in 15-minute increments.

D9970. Enamel microabrasion.

The removal of discolored surface enamel defects resulting from altered mineralization or decalcification of the superficial enamel layer. Submit per treatment visit.

Source: CDT® 2011–2012, *The ADA® Practical Guide to Dental Procedure Codes Book*

Children and Caries, Specific Recommendations for Ages 0–5

Early childhood caries has increased significantly in children, particularly those aged 2–5 years.[94] The disease progression in this age group has been the subject of numerous recent headline media reports. Caries Management by Risk Assessment (CAMBRA) is recommended by the American Academy of Pediatric Dentistry as a primary method of intervention and education. Many parents and caregivers are unaware of several important issues regarding the dental caries risk of children. For example, caregivers play a role in the bacterial transmission to their child. Caregivers pass organisms and bacterial species responsible for dental decay through close contact and the sharing of saliva in a process termed vertical transmission.[95] Caregivers are often surprised to learn that there are specific risks associated with childhood caries and that therapy recommendations made in order to lower the child's risk and symptoms of dental disease include home care therapy recommendations for the caregiver as well.[96] Furthermore, during pregnancy, women often fail to recognize the critical importance good oral health and regular dental visits may have on the long-term oral health of their children.[97]

CAMBRA is designed to systematically assess each child's and their caregiver's caries risks, tailor a specific therapeutic management plan in conjunction with a restorative plan, and provide guidance for appropriate periodic reassessment based on the individual risk of the patient.[98] Due to the speed with which children and their habits change between the ages of 0 and 5, risk assessment should be performed at an initial appointment as well as at all subsequent appointments. While the evidence and effectiveness of preventive and treatment methods continues to grow, children's risks and specific needs differ widely and standardized protocols are limited.[98] Therefore, both patients and practitioners should expect to modify the patients' caries therapy plan regularly based on risk and therapies available.

In order to prevent and manage the disease, it is recommended that dental visits begin early, and children should have a comprehensive oral exam by age 1.[97] During the exam, the practitioner performs a caries risk assessment, looking specifically at risk factors for the disease, bacterial biofilm challenge (if applicable), and disease indicators. Dental exams for children are similar to those experienced by adults, and there are five straightforward steps involved.

Step 1. Through a short interview with the caregiver, the practitioner gathers information regarding the child's specific risk factors for the disease. Risk factors for the disease include those risk factors already discussed for adults, but other risk factors specific to children are also assessed. At this time, if applicable, a bacterial screening test is also performed to assess the patient's and the caregiver's bacterial biofilm challenges.

Step 2. The practitioner then performs a prophylaxis cleaning of the child's teeth and possibly demonstrates proper cleaning techniques for the caregiver.

Step 3. The dentist then performs a clinical examination. During the examination, the dentist looks for disease indicators such as current decay, white spot lesions, decalcifications of the enamel, or the presence of restorations indicating past caries experience.

Step 4. Based on the patient's caries risk assessment, the ADA recommends that a fluoride varnish be applied every 3 to 6 months to help prevent decay.[94]

Step 5. Based on the risk assessment and clinical examination, the caregiver and the dental professional work to determine mutually agreed-upon oral health goals for the child and the family. Ideally, one or two home management goals are established for reassessment at the next appointment to reduce the risk factors for dental disease and increase the protective factors.

Risk Factors for Ages 0–5

In order to identify if a child is at risk for cavities, the caregiver and the dental practitioner must identify if the child has any risk factors for the disease. A risk factor is simply something that increases the child's risk for a disease.

Because children may have very little dental history due to their age, risk factors by themselves can place a child at high risk for dental decay. The best method of lowering a child's caries risk is to reduce any and all modifiable risk factors. If unmodifiable risk factors exist, or patients would prefer, professional/prescription home care therapy products should be dispensed.

Risk Factors for Children Aged 0–5[96, 98]

Elevated levels of ATP by CariScreen and/or cavity-causing bacteria by culture.

Mother/caregiver(s) has elevated levels of ATP as determined by CariScreen.

Mother/Caregiver(s) has had dental decay in the last 12 months (family history of decay).

Takes bottle or drinks liquid *other than* water or milk/formula/breastfed.

Frequent/continual bottles/drinks other than water.

Child sleeps with bottle/drinks other than water or nurses on demand.

Frequent snacking between meals (three or more times daily other than meals).

Saliva-reducing factors present (medications, medical condition, genetic factors).

Cariogenic diet (sugars, sugared/acidic beverages, starch foods, fermentable carbohydrates).

Child has developmental problems (special needs).

Low socioeconomic status and/or caregiver has low health literacy.

Disease Indicators for Ages 0–5[96, 98]

Disease indicators are signs and symptoms of the disease, and the presence of one disease indicator places the child at high risk, and based on the risk factors present, professional / prescription therapy should be dispensed.

Current decay, white spot lesions, decalcification / defects of the enamel.

Restorations present (past caries / decay experience).

Plaque is obvious on teeth or gums bleed easily.

Visually inadequate saliva flow.

Risk Categories for Ages 0–5 (Per ADA Caries Risk Criteria)[96,98]

Low caries risk.
Patient has zero risk factors and no decay in the last 3 years.

Moderate caries risk.
Patient has one risk factor and no decay in the last 3 years.

High risk or high/extreme caries risk.
Patient has two or more risk factors and/or decay in the last 3 years.

Therapy Recommendations for Ages 0–5[96, 98]

Low Risk

Low-risk patients' caregivers should be aware of the risks associated with dental disease and share the information with other family members and caregivers, maintaining good home care habits with preventive dental care products such as tooth wipes for infants and toddlers and gels and sprays for all ages. Preventive products should contain pH neutralization, xylitol, and remineralization agents such as nanohydroxyapatite whenever possible. The dental practitioner will advise on the use of fluoride-containing oral care products based on the age and risk of the child. Caregivers should be aware if they live in a water-fluoridated community as drinking fluoridated water is a protective factor.

Moderate Risk

Moderate risk patients' caregivers should be aware of the risks associated with dental disease and share the information with other family members and caregivers. If possible, caregivers should consider the benefit of eliminating the risk factor placing the child at risk. Maintaining good home care habits with preventive dental care products such as tooth wipes for infants and toddlers and gels and sprays for all ages. Preventive products should contain pH neutralization, xylitol, and remineralization agents such as nanohydroxyapatite whenever possible. The dental practitioner will advise on the use of fluoride-containing oral care products based on the age and risk of the child. Caregivers should be aware if they live in a water-fluoridated community as drinking fluoridated water is a protective factor.

High Risk

High-risk patients' caregivers should be aware of the risks associated with dental disease and share the information with other family members and caregivers. If possible, caregivers should consider the benefit of eliminating the risk factor(s) placing the child at risk. For high-risk patients aged 0–2, caregivers should brush the child's teeth / gums at least 2 times daily with a gel that contains pH neutralization, xylitol, and nanoparticles of hydroxyapatite. Such products are safe to swallow. Caregivers should also use xylitol wipes infused with pH neutralization 3–4 times daily after every meal / bottle. Based on the clinician's judgment, a small smear of gel that contains a small amount of fluoride can be used along with pH neutralization, xylitol, and nanoparticles of hydroxyapatite as a toothpaste replacement for the gel which does not contain fluoride.[96] Use caution when using fluoride products on infants and toddlers. A smear of gel with pH neutralization, xylitol, and nanoparticles of hydroxyapatite should also be applied and left on at bedtime.[96] Fluoride varnish should be performed at initial dental visits and at 3-month recalls.

Caregivers of patients aged 0–2 should also consider adding products with 0.05% neutral sodium fluoride, antibacterials (0.2% sodium hypochlorite), pH neutralization, and xylitol, along with toothpaste/gel with pH neutralization, fluoride (1.1% NaF), xylitol, and nanoparticles of hydroxyapatite to their home care regimen. A change to professional/prescription home care therapy products for the caregiver(s) may reduce the risk of vertical transmission of the cavity-causing bacterial species.[96]

High-risk patients' caregivers should be aware of the risks associated with dental disease and share the information with other family members and caregivers. If possible, caregivers should consider the benefit of eliminating the risk factor(s) placing the child at risk. For high-risk patients aged 3–5, caregivers should brush the patients' teeth/gums at least 2 times daily with a small smear of gel that contains a small amount of fluoride (0.243%), along with pH neutralization, xylitol, and nanoparticles of hydroxyapatite as a toothpaste. Use caution when using fluoride products on infants and toddlers. Caregivers should also use oral wipes and mouth sprays infused with xylitol and pH neutralization, 3–4 times daily after every meal/bottle. A smear of gel with pH neutralization, xylitol, and nanoparticles of hydroxyapatite should also be applied and left on at bedtime.[96] Fluoride varnish should be performed at initial dental visits and recalls.[44]

Caregivers of patients aged 3–5 should also consider adding products such as 0.05% neutral sodium fluoride, antibacterials (0.2% sodium hypochlorite), pH neutralization, and xylitol, along with toothpaste/gel with pH neutralization, fluoride (1.1% NaF), xylitol, and nanoparticles of hydroxyapatite, to their home care regimen. A change to professional/prescription home care therapy products with xylitol for the caregiver(s) may reduce the risk of vertical transmission of the cavity-causing bacterial species.[96]

Other Recommendations

Depending on the severity of the patient's risk and the clinical judgment of the dentist, some clinicians have also added additional recommendations to those above for children aged 3–5. The FDA recommends that all 0.05% neutral sodium fluoride rinses be prescribed only to children aged 6 and up.[99] Antibacterial rinses such as the 0.2% sodium hypochlorite and 0.05% fluoride also fall under this category. But for children that are capable of rinsing and spitting, some practitioners have recommended adding such rinses for a patient in the 3–5 age group home care regimen. In order to reduce the risk of swallowing, it is sometimes recommended that the caregiver brush the rinse on with a toothbrush and have the child spit every 5 to 10 seconds. Clinicians will only make these types of other recommendations when they feel the benefit outweighs the risk. Children that have had to undergo anesthesia in a hospital setting in order to have dental treatment due to decay may fit this category.

Sealants

Clinicians should follow all ADA and AAPD guidelines on sealants, and glass ionomer–based materials are recommended on all deep pits and fissures. [96]

What about Probiotics?

Due to the role bacterial biofilms play in the dental caries process, interest and research in probiotics has accelerated. Some products that are currently on the market and contain bacterial species such as *Streptococcus oralis*, *Streptococcus uberis*, *Streptococcus rattus*, and forms of *Lactobacillus* and *Bifidobacteria* are being researched. While these species of bacteria are generally recognized as safe for human consumption, results from meta-analyses and systematic reviews that combine results of studies from different types of probiotics to examine the effects in any disease state should be interpreted with caution. In isolated studies, some specific probiotic strains have been shown to be effective in specific disease states under certain conditions. However, no two probiotics are exactly alike; and professionals should not expect reproducible results from studies that employ different species or strains, variable formulations, and diverse dosing schedules.[100] Until further research is performed regarding probiotics, clinicians and patients should focus on creating a healthy oral environment by neutralizing the pH and supporting the patient's natural healthy oral microflora.

When a patient's oral environment is out of balance, and the biofilm has converted to primarily aciduric cariogenic species, healthy bacteria are unable to survive.[19] Unless the pH dysfunction is corrected, the introduction of "probiotic" species is unlikely have a sustainable effect on the biofilm makeup. As demonstrated earlier in the studies conducted by the authors using PCR and 16S gene sequencing DNA identification, when the pH of the oral environment is altered using pH neutralization and/or antibacterials such as 0.2% sodium hypochlorite, the patient's natural healthy oral microflora returns. This data demonstrates that the addition of probiotics is not required for healthy biofilm conversion. Conversely, if the pH dysfunction is not addressed, natural healthy oral bacterial species, whether introduced naturally or by probiotic products, may not survive and therefore cannot sustainably alter the oral biofilm toward health. A patient's oral biofilm makeup is as specific to them as their fingerprint and probiotic bacterial species may not be a sustainable member of each and every patient's natural healthy biofilm community. Research continues to explore the role probiotics may play in treating this disease in the future.

What about Chlorhexidine for Caries Treatment?

Chlorhexidine rinse has been prescribed routinely in the past for dental caries therapy. But recently, studies have demonstrated that caries preventive therapy with CHX resulted in population increases of highly acidogenic or acid-tolerant *MS* strains. The implications are that caries preventive therapy may not always eliminate *MS* strains with cariogenic potential and, in fact, may select for the survival of the most pathogenic phylotype of *MS*.[101] Furthermore, in a recent publication in the *Journal of the American Dental Association* in April 2011, the ADA Council on Scientific Affairs reviewed evidence from 50 randomized controlled trials and 15 nonrandomized studies to assess the efficacy of various nonfluoride caries-preventive agents. In the results, the ADA Council on Scientific Affairs stated that beyond CHX-thymol varnish every 3 months for root surface lesions, all other CHX products in any form, for any lesion site, for any age, is *not recommended*.[102]

Can It Be Done?

Thousands of dental practices and millions of patients in the United States have seen the benefits of CAMBRA methodologies. Dental caries is still an epidemic in the United States; and this book was prepared with the guidance of expert individuals, hygienists, dentists, and dental professors with the goal of educating and providing both patients and practitioners a guide for reducing dental decay and improving oral health. It can be done. It is being done!

Disclaimer

Every effort has been made to ensure that the information provided in this book is accurate, up-to-date, and complete; but no guarantee is made to that effect. In addition, the information contained herein may be time sensitive. This information does not endorse drugs, diagnose patients, or recommend therapy. It is a reference resource designed as supplement to, and not a substitute for, the expertise, skills, knowledge, and judgment of health care practitioners in patient care. The absence of a warning for a given drug or drug combination in no way should be construed to indicate that the drug or drug combination is safe, effective, or appropriate for any given patient. The authors do not assume any responsibility for any aspect of health care administered with the aid of information this book provides. The information contained herein is not intended to cover all possible uses, directions, precautions, warnings, drug interactions, allergic reactions, and adverse effects. If you have questions, check with your dentist, hygienist, doctor, nurse, or pharmacist.

Handbook References

1. *Oral Health America: A Report of the US Surgeon General* 63 (2000): 79–94, 245.

2. National Institute of Health, US Dept. of Health and Human Services, "Diagnosis and Management of Dental Caries throughout Life" 18, no. 1 (March 2001).

3. O. Fejerskov and E. Kidd, *Dental Caries: The Disease and Its Clinical Management* (Oxford, UK: Blackwell Munksgaard, 2003), 4–5.

4. D. A. Young, V. K. Kutsch, and J. Whitehouse, "A Clinician's Guide to CAMBRA: A Simple Approach," *Compend Contin Educ Dent* 30, no. 2 (2009): 92–98.

5. D. A. Young, J. D. Featherstone, J. R. Roth, M. Anderson, J. Autio-Gold, G. J. Christensen, M. Fontana, V. K. Kutsch, M. C. Peters, R. J. Simonsen, and M. S. Wolff, "Caries Management by Risk Assessment: Implementation Guidelines," *J Calif Dent Assoc* 35, no. 11 (Nov. 2007): 799–805.

6. J. D. B. Featherstone, "The Science and Practice of Caries Prevention," *J Am Dent Assoc* 131, no. 7 (2000): 887–899.

7. V. Uskokovic´, W. Li, and S. Habelitz, "Amelogenin as a Promoter of Nucleation and Crystal Growth of Apatite," *J of Crystal Growth* 316, no. 1 (2011): 106–117.

8. J. D. B. Featherstone, J. M. White, C. I. Hoover, M. Rapozo-Hilo, J. A. Weintraub, R. S. Wilson, L. Zhan, and S. A. Gansky, "A Randomized Clinical Trial of Anticaries Therapies Targeted according to Risk Assessment (Caries Management by Risk Assessment)," *Caries Res* 46 (2012): 118–129.

9. O. Fejerskov and E. Kidd, *Dental Caries: The Disease and Its Clinical Management* (Oxford, UK: Blackwell Munksgaard, 2003).

10. H. J. Busscher and L. V. Evan, *Oral Biofilms and Plaque Control* (Amsterdam, the Netherlands: Harwood Academic Publishers, 1998).

11. K. Nakano, H. Nemoto, R. Nomura, H. Inaba, H. Yoshioka, K. Taniguchi, A. Amano, and T. Ooshima, "Detection of Oral Bacteria in Cardiovascular Specimens," *Oral MicrobiolImmunol* 24, no. 1 (2009): 64–68.

12. J. Abranches, J. H. Miller, A. R. Martinez, P. J. Simpson-Haidaris, R. A. Burne, and J. A. Lemos. "The Collagen-Binding Protein Cnm Is Required for *Streptococcus mutans* Adherence to and Intracellular Invasion of Human Coronary Artery Endothelial Cells," *Infect Immun* 79, no. 6 (June 2011): 2277–84.

13. A. Kojima, K. Nakano, et al., "Infection of Specific Strains of *Streptococcus mutans*, Oral Bacteria, Confers a Risk of Ulcerative Colitis," *Sci Rep* 2 (2012): 332.

14. S. K. Filoche, D. Soma, M. van Bekkum, and C. H. Sissons, "Plaques from Different Individuals Yields Different Microbiota Responses to Oral-Antiseptic Treatment," *FEMS Immunol Med Microbiol* 54 (2008): 27–36.

15. R.A. Bagramian, F. Garcia-Godoy, and A. R. Volpe, "The Global Increase in Dental Caries: A Pending Public Health Crisis," *Am J Dent* 22, no. 1 (February 2009): 3–8.

16. A. C. Tanner, J. M. Mathney, R. L. Kent Jr., et al., "Cultivable Anaerobic Microbiota of Severe Early Childhood Caries," *J ClinMicrobiol* 49, no. 4 (April 2011): 1464–74.

17. V. K. Kutsch, C. L. Kutsch, and B. C. Nelson, "A Clinical Look at CAMBRA," *DPR* 41, no. 8 (August 2007): 62–67.

18. N. Takahashi and B. Nyvad, "The Role of Bacteria in the Caries Process: Ecological Perspectives," *J Dent Res* 90, no. 3 (March 2011): 294–303.

19. P. D. Marsh, "Dental Plaque as a Biofilm: The Significance of pH in Health and Caries," *CompendContinEduc Dent* 30, no. 2 (March 2009): 76–8.

20. N. Takahashi and B. Nyvad, "The Role of Bacteria in the Caries Process: Ecological Perspectives," *JDR* 90, no. 3 (March 2011): 294–303.

21. P. E. Kolenbrander, "Oral Microbial Communities: Biofilms, Interactions, and Genetic Systems," *Annul Rev Microbiol* 54 (2000): 413–437.

22. O. Fejerskov, and E. Kidd, *Dental Caries: The Disease and Its Clinical Management* (Oxford, UK: Blackwell Munksgaard, 2003), 4–5.

23. Sophie Domejean, Joel M White, and John D. B. Featherstone, "Validation of the CDA CAMBRA Caries Risk Assessment —A Six-Year Retrospective Study," *J Calif Dent Assoc* 39, no. 10 (2011): 709–15.

24. B. Rosan, R. J. Lamont, "Dental Plaque Formation," *Microbes Infect* 2 (2000): 1599–607.

25. Y. Li, Y. Ge, D. Saxena, and P. W Caufield, "Genetic Profiling of the Oral Microbia Associated with Severe Early-Childhood Caries," *J Clinical Microbiology* 45, no. 1 (January 2007): 81–87.

26. S. Matthijs, M. M. Sabzevar, and P.A. Adriaens, "Intra-Examiner Reproducibility of 4 Dental Plaque Indices," *J ClinPeriodontol* 28, no.3 (Mrach 2001): 250–4.

27. Leo M. Sreebny and Arjan Vissink, *Dry Mouth, the Malevolent Symptom* (Hoboken, NJ: Wiley-Blackwell, 2010), 12, fig. 1.2.2.

28. V. K. Kutsch and C. Cady, "MIX Disease: Diagnosis and Treatment," *Inside Dentistry* 5, no. 7 (2009): 80–83.

29. http://www.ada.org/sections/newsAndEvents/pdfs/ltr_dry_mouth_110427.pdf.

30. Leo M. Sreebny and ArjanVissink, *Dry Mouth, the Malevolent Symptom* (Hoboken, NJ: Wiley-Blackwell, 2010), 98.

31. *AGD Dry Mouth Brochure*, http://www.agd.org/public/OralHealth/drymouth/Dry_Mouth_Brochure.pdf.

32. Leo M. Sreebny and ArjanVissink, *Dry Mouth, the Malevolent Symptom* (Hoboken, NJ: Wiley-Blackwell, 2010), 92.

33. John D. B. Featherstone, Sophie Domejean-Orliaguet, Larry Jenson, Mark Wolff, and Douglas A. Young, "Caries Risk Assessment in Practice Ages 6 Through Adult," *J Calif Dent Assoc* 35, no. 10 (2007): 703–13.

34. M. Enaia, N. Bock, and S. Ruf, "White-Spot Lesions during Multibracket Appliance Treatment: A Challenge for Clinical Excellence," *Am J OrthodDentofacialOrthop* 140, no. 1 (July 2011): e17–24.

35. Philip D. Marsh, Michael V. Martin, *Oral Microbiology*, 5th ed. (2009), 15–16.

36. P. D. Marsh, "Dental Plaque as a Biofilm and a Microbial Community—Implications for Health and Disease," *BMC Oral Health* 6, Suppl. 1 (2006): S14.

37. G. Topping and A. Assaf, "Strong Evidence That Daily Use of Fluoride Toothpaste Prevents Caries," *Evid Based Dent* 6, no. 2 (2005): 32.

38. American Academy of Pediatric Dentistry Council on Clinical Affairs, "Guideline on Infant Oral Health Care," *AAPD Reference Manual* 33 (2011): 6–11/12.

39. J. M. Ten Cate and J. D. Featherstone, "Mechanistic Aspects of the Interactions between Fluoride and Dental Enamel," *Crit Rev Oral Biol Med* 2, no. 3 (1991): 283–96.

40. J. D. Featherstone, R. Glena, M. Shariati, and C. P. Shields, "Dependence of In Vitro Demineralization of Apatite and Remineralization of Dental Enamel on Fluoride Concentration," *J Dent Res* 69 (1990): 620–625.

41. A. Dasanayake and P. W. Caufield, "At-Home or In-Office Fluoride Application Does Not Significantly Reduce Subsequent Caries-Related Procedures in Ambulatory Adults of Any Caries-Risk Level," *J Evid Base Dent Practice* 7 (2007): 155–157.

42. H. Maehara, Y. Iwami, H. Mayanagi, and N. Takahashi, "Synergistic Inhibition by Combination of Fluoride and Xylitol on Glycolysis by *Mutans streptococci* and Its Biochemical Mechanism, *Caries Res* 39, no. 6 (2005): 521–528.

43. J. F. McClendon, C. W. Foster, Ludwick, and J. C. Criswell "Delay of Dental Caries by Fluorine," *J Dent Res* 21, no. 2 (April 1942): 139–143.

44. J. L. Sintes, C. Escalante, B. Stewart, et al., "Enhanced Anticaries Efficacy of a 0.243% Sodium Fluoride / 10% Xylitol / Silica Dentifrice: 3 Year Clinical Results," *Am J Dent* 8, no. 5 (1995): 231–5.

45. J. L. Sintes, A. Elias-Boneta, B. Stewart, et al., "Anticaries Efficacy of a Sodium Monofluorophosphate Dentifrice Containing Xylitol in a Dicalcium Phosphate Dihydrate Base: A 30 Month Caries Clinical Study in Costa Rica," *Am J Dent* 15, no. 4 (2002): 215–9.

46. P. L. Phillips, R. D. Wolcott, J. Fletcher, and G.S. Schultz, "Biofilms Made Easy," *Wnds Intl* 1, no. 3 (May 2010).

47. H. Cho, H. Jönsson, K. Campbell, P. Melke, J. W. Williams, B. Jedynak, et al., "http://www.agd.org/public/OralHealth/drymouth/Dry_Mouth_Brochure.pdf," *PLoS Biology* 5, no. 11 (2007): e302 EP.

48. http://www.biofilm.montana.edu/

49. D. M. Winn, W. J. Blot, J. K. McLaughlin, et al., "Mouthwash Use and Oral Conditions in the Risk of Oral and Pharyngeal Cancer," *Cancer Research* 51 (1991): 3044–3047.

50. C . W. Werner and R. A. Seymour, "Are Alcohol Containing Mouthwashes Safe?" *British Dental Journal* 207 (2009): E19.

51. M. J. McCullough and C. S. Farah, "The Role of Alcohol in Oral Carcinogenesis with Particular Reference to Alcohol-Containing Mouthwashes," *Aust Dent J* 53 (2008): 302–305.

52. A. L. Boskey and A. S. Posner, "Conversion of Amorphous Calcium Phosphate to Microcrystalline Hydroxyapatite: A pH Dependent, Solution Mediated, Solid-Solid Conversion," *Journal of Physical Chemistry* 77, no. 19 (1973): 2313.

53. R. Štulajterová and L. Medveckýa, "Effect of Calcium Ions on Transformation Brushite to Hydroxyapatite in Aqueous Solutions," *Colloids and Surfaces A: Physicochemical and Engineering Aspects* 316, no. 1 (2008): 104–109.

54. R. L. Karlinsey, A. C. Mackey, E. R. Walker, and K. E. Frederick, "Surfactant-Modified ß-TCP: Structure, Properties, and In Vitro Remineralization of Subsurface Enamel Lesions," *J Mater Sci* 21 (2010): 2009–2020.

55. R. L. Karlinsey, A. C. Mackey, G. K. Stookey, and A. M. Pfarrer, In Vitro Assessments of Experimental NaF Dentifrices Containing a Prospective Calcium Phosphate Technology," *Am J Dent* 22 (2009): 180–184.

56. E. C. Reynolds, "Casein Phosphopeptide-Amorphous Calcium Phosphate: The Scientific Evidence," *Adv Dent Res* 21 (2009): 25–29.

57. A. Azarpazhooh and H. Limeback, "Clinical efficacy of Casein Derivatives: A Systematic Review of the Literature," *J Am Dent Assoc* 139 (2008): 915–924.

58. M. V. Morgan, G. G. Adams, D. L. Bailey, C. E. Tsao, S. L. Fischman, and E. C. Reynolds, "The Anticariogenic Effect of Sugar-Free Gum Containing CPP-ACP Nanocomplexes on Approximal Caries Determined Using Digital Bitewing Radiography," *Caries Res* 42 (2008): 171–184.

59. S. Lata, N. O. Varghese, and Jolly Mary Varughese, "Remineralization potential of fluoride and Amorphous Calcium Phosphate-Casein Phospho Peptide on Enamel Lesions: An In Vitro Comparative Evaluation," *J Conserv Dent* 13, no. 1 (2010): 42–46.

60. L. J. Walsh, "Evidence That Demands a Verdict: Latest Developments in Remineralization Therapies," *Australasian Dental Practice* (March/April2009): 48–59.

61. T. Tanaka, N. Yagi, T. Ohta, Y. Matsuo, H. Terada, K. Kamasaka, K. To-o, T. Komentani, and T. Kuriki, "Evaluation of the Distribution and Orientation of Remineralized Enamel Crystallites in Subsurface Lesions by X-ray Diffraction," *Caries Res* 44, no. 3 (2010): 253–9.

62. R. Takikawa, K. Fujitsu, T. Ishizaki, and R. E. Hayman, "Restoration of Post-bleach Enamel Gloss Using a Non-abrasive, Nano-hydroxyapatite Conditioner," *J Dent Res* Special Issue B (Brsibane Abstracts; 2006): 85.

63. S. B. Huang, S. S. Gao, and H. Y. Yu, "Effect of Nano-hydroxyapatite Concentration on Remineralization of Initial Enamel Lesion In Vitro," *Biomed Mater* 4, no. 3 (2009): 034104.

64. L. Li, H. Pan, J. Tao, X. Xu, C. Mao, X. Gu, and R. Tang, "Repair of Enamel by Using Hydroxyapatite Nanoparticles as the Building Blocks," *J of Mater Chem* 18 (2008): 4079–4084.

65. R. P. Allaker, "The Use of Nanoparticles to Control Oral Biofilm Formation," *J Dent Res* 89, no. 11 (2010): 1175–1186.

66. R. Asa, "Proactive Prevention: Treating Caries Disease with Remineralization," *AGD Impact Journal* 39, no. 2 (February 2011): 20–24.

67. N. Roveri, E. Battistella, C. L. Bianchi, et al., "Surface Enamel Remineralization: Biomimetic Apatite Nanocrystals and Fluoride Ions Different Effects," *J of Nanomaterials* (2009): 1–9.

68. Based on a private practice study of 3,125 patients, http://carifree.com/dentist/learn/our-systems/data-study.html

69. N. B. Pitts and P. A. Rimmer, "An In Vivo Comparison of Radiographic and Directly Assessed Clinical Caries Status of Posterior Approximal Surfaces in Primary and Permanent Teeth," *Caries Res* 26 (1992): 146–152.

70. E. Theilade, O. Fejerskov, T. Karring, and J. Theilade, "Predominantecultivalemicroflora of Human Dental Fissure Plaque," *Infect Immun* 36, no. 3 (1982): 977–982.

71. P. Arneberg, B. Ogaard, A. A. Scheie, and G. Rolla, "Selection of *Streptococcus mutans* and *Lactobacilli* in an Intra-oral Human Caries Model," *J Dent Res* 63, no. 10 (1984): 1197–1200.

72. D. Boue, E. Armau, and G. Tiraby, "A Bacteriological Study of Rampant Caries in Children," *J Dent Res* 66 1 (1987): 23–28.

73. B. Kohler and S. Bjarnason, "*Mutans streptococci*, *Lactobacilli* and Caries Prevalence in 11 and 12-Year-Old Icelandic Children," *Community Dent Oral Epidemiol* 15, no. 6 (1987): 52–55.

74. V. K. Kutsch, C. L. Kutsch, and B. C. Nelson, "A Clinical Look at CAMBRA," *Dental Products Report* 41, no. 8 (2007): 62–67.

75. M. A. Munson, A. Banerjee, T. F. Watson, and W. G. Wade, Molecular Analysis of the Microflora Associated with Dental Caries," *J ClinMicrobiol* 42, no. 7 (2004): 3023–3029.

76. M. R. Becker, B. J. Paster, E. J. Leys, et al., "Molecular Analysis of Bacterial Species Associated with Childhood Caries," *J ClinMicrobiol* 40, no. 3 (2002): 1001–1009.

77. D. Beighton, "The Complex Oral Microflora of High-Risk Individuals and Groups and Its Role in the Caries Process," *Community Dent Oral Epidemiol* 5, no. 4 (2005): 248–255.

78. J. vanHoute, J. Lopman, and R. Kent, "The Predominant Cultivable Flora of Sound and Carious Human Root Surfaces," *J Dent Res* 73, no. 11 (1994): 1727–1734.

79. M. L. Hayes and A. M. Acevedo, "Microbiological Composition of Dental Plaque from Different Areas of the Mouth," *ActaOdontol Venez* 25, no. 2 (1987): 223–240.

80. W. J. Loesche, "Role of *Streptococcus mutans* in Human Dental Decay," *Microbiol Review* 50, no. 4 (1986): 353–380.

81. T. Hamada, H. Nikawa, H. Yamashiro, et al., "In Vitro Cariogenic Potential of *Candida albicans*," *Mycoses* 46, no. 11–12 (2003): 471–478.

82. I. Kleinberg, "A Mixed-Bacteria Ecological Approach to Understanding the Role of Bacteria in Dental Caries Causation: An Alternative to *Streptococcus mutans* and the Specific Plaque Hypothesis," *Critical Reviews in Oral Biology and Medicine* 13 (2002): 108–125.

83. H. K. Yip, J. H. Guo, and W. H. Wong, "Incipient Caries Lesions on Cementum by Mono and Co-culture Oral Bacteria," *J Dent* 35, no. 5 (2007): 377–382.

84. A. C. Tanner, P. M. Milgrom, R. Kent Jr., et al., "The Microbiota of Young Children from Tooth and Tongue Samples," *J Dent Res* 81, no. 1 (2002): 53–57.

85. E. Hoshino, "Predominant Obligate Anaerobes in Human Carious Dentin," *J Dent Res* 64, no. 10 (1985): 1195–8.

86. C. H. Sissons, S. A. Anderson, L. Wong, et al., "Microbiota of Plaque Biofilms: Effect of Three Times Daily Sucrose Pulses in Different Simulated Oral Environments," *Caries Res* 41, no. 5 (2007): 413–422.

87. J. A. Aas, A. L. Griffen, S. R. Dardis, et al., "Bacteria of Dental Caries in Primary and Permanent Teeth in Children and Young Adults," *J ClinMicrobiol* 46, no. 4 (2008): 1407–1417.

88. D. Preza, I. Olsen, J. A. Aas, et al., "Bacterial Profiles of Root Caries in Elderly Patients," *J ClinMicrobiol* 46, no. 6 (2008): 2015–2021.

89. N. Takahashi and B. Nyvad, "Caries Ecology Revisited: Microbial Dynamics and the Caries Process," *Caries Res* 42, no. 6 (2008): 409–418.

90. M. Wilson, *Microbial Inhabitants of Humans* (Cambridge Press Publishers, 2005), 59–352.

91. Y. Li, Y. Ge, D. Saxena, and P. W. Caufield, "Genetic Profiling of the Oral Microbia Associated with Severe Early-Childhood Caries," *J Clin Micro* 45, no. 1 (2007): 81–87.

92. R. Sauerwein, P. Pellegrini, J. Finlayson, et al., *ATP Bioluminescence: Quantitative Assessment of Plaque Bacteria Surrounding Orthodontic Appliances* (Portland, OR: Oregon Health and Science University, 2008) IADR Abstract no. 1288.

93. Alice C. L. Len, D. W. S. Harty, and A. J. Jaques, "Stress-Responsive Proteins Are Upregulated in *Streptococcus mutans* during Acid Tolerance," *Microbiol* 150 (2004): 159–1351.

94. B. A. Dye, O. Arevalo, and C. M. Vargas, "Trends in Pediatric Dental Caries by Poverty Status in the United States, 1988–1997 and 1994–2004," *Int J Paediatric Dent* 20, no. 2 (2010): 132–43.

95. American Academy of Pediatric Dentistry, "Policy on the Dental Home," *AAPD Reference Manual* 31, no. 6: 22–3.

96. Francisco Ramos-Gomez and Man-Wai Ng, "Into the Future: Keeping Healthy Teeth Caries Free: Pediatric CAMBRA Protocols," *J Calif Dent Assoc* 39, no. 10 (2011): 723–33.

97. S. Gajendra and J. V. Kumar, "Oral Health and Pregnancy: A Review," *NY State Dent J* 70, no. 1 (2004):40–4.

98. American Dental Association Council on Scientific Affairs, "Professionally Applied Topical Fluoride: Evidence-Based Clinical Recommendations," *JADA* 137, no. 8 (August 2006): 1151–1159.

99. "Anticaries Drug Products for Over-the-Counter Human Use," *Code of Federal Regulations*, title 21, vol. 5, 21 CFR 355.

100. A. Minocha, "Probiotics for Preventive Health," *NutrClinPract* 24, no. 2 (April–May 2009): 227–41.

101. E. Palmer, T. Finlayson, T. Nielsen, et al., "Selection of *Mutans streptococci* Strains Following Caries Preventive Therapy," *AADR* (2010): Abstract #.

102. M. P. Rethman, E. D. Beltran-Aguilar, R. J. Billings, et al., "Nonfluoride Caries-Preventive Agents: Executive Summary of Evidence-Based Clinical Recommendations," *JADA* 142, no. 9 (September 2011): 1065–71.

About the Authors

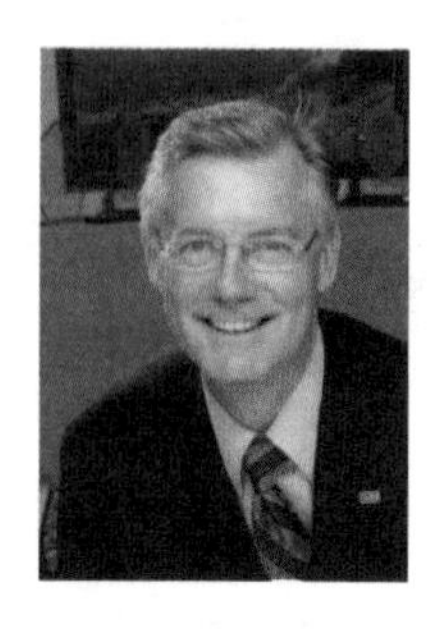

V. Kim Kutsch, DMD, received his undergraduate degree from the Westminster College in Utah and then completed his DMD at the University of Oregon School of Dentistry in 1979. He is an inventor (holding numerous patents in dentistry), product consultant, internationally recognized speaker, past president of the Academy of Laser Dentistry and the World Congress of Minimally Invasive Dentistry. He has also served on the board of directors for the *World Clinical Laser Institute* and the *American Academy of Cosmetic Dentistry*. As an author, Dr. Kutsch has published dozens of articles and abstracts on minimally invasive dentistry, caries risk assessment, digital radiography, and other technologies in both dental and medical journals and has also contributed in several textbooks. He acts as a reviewer for several journals including the *Journal of the American Dental Association*. He serves as CEO of Oral BioTech. As a clinician, he is a graduate and mentor in the prestigious Kois Center and maintains a private practice in Albany, Oregon.

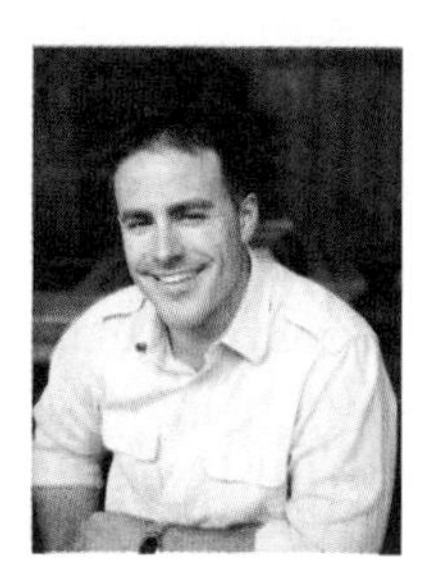

Robert J. Bowers obtained a Bachelor of Science in Business Management Information Systems with a minor in Economics from Oregon State University. With over twelve years of experience in dental manufacturing and dental systems design, he has played an integral role in building dental preventive care models. Bob is an inventor currently holding multiple dental-related patents. He has invented and introduced a number of caries treatment products and protocols within the dental industry. Bob has participated with the CAMBRA Coalition in furthering the field of caries risk assessment in dentistry. He has worked with over 5,000 dental practices in implementing caries risk assessment methods and standards and has designed CAMBRA systems and products currently used in dental schools across the United States. Bob currently serves as the Chief Operating Officer of Oral BioTech.

To learn more visit
www.balancebook.com